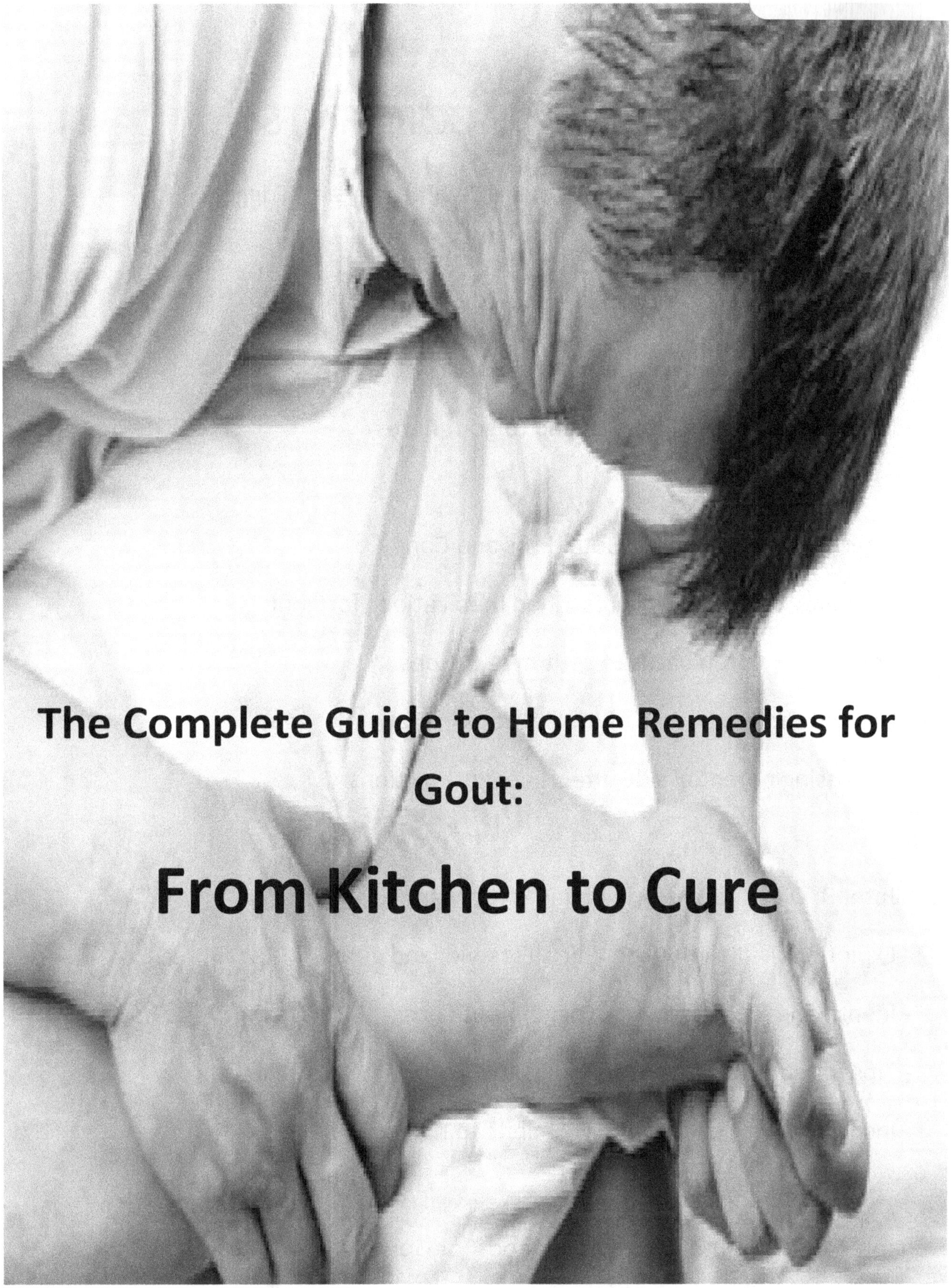

The Complete Guide to Home Remedies for Gout:

From Kitchen to Cure

TABLE OF CONTENTS

- Different ways to incorporate apple cider vinegar into daily routine

- Precautions and potential side effects

Chapter 12: Cherry Juice and Gout: Does it Really Help?

- Investigating the connection between cherry juice and gout relief

- Analyzing scientific evidence supporting its efficacy

- Exploring the potential mechanisms behind cherry juice's benefits

- Recommendations for incorporating cherry juice into a gout management plan

Chapter 13: Turmeric and Ginger for Gout: Spicing Up Your Health

- Overview of turmeric and ginger and their anti-inflammatory properties

- Discussing their potential benefits for gout management

- Methods of incorporating turmeric and ginger into meals and beverages

- Precautions and considerations for using these spices

Chapter 14: The Magic of Epsom Salt for Gout Pain Relief

- Understanding the role of Epsom salt in gout relief

- Exploring its potential benefits for reducing pain and inflammation

- Different ways to use Epsom salt baths or compresses for gout relief

- Safety precautions and considerations when using Epsom salt

- Tips for maintaining a healthy weight and managing comorbidities

- Resources for ongoing support and self-care in gout management

Conclusion: Achieving Gout Relief Through Home Remedies

- Recap of key takeaways from the book

- Encouragement for incorporating home remedies into a comprehensive gout management plan

- Empowering readers to take control of their gout and improve their quality of life

Introduction:

Welcome to "The Complete Guide to Home Remedies for Gout: From Kitchen to Cure." In the following pages, we embark on a journey of understanding and empowerment for those seeking relief from the painful grip of gout. This comprehensive guide is designed to provide you with a wealth of knowledge, practical tips and effective home remedies to help you manage and relieve your gout symptoms.

Gout, a form of arthritis, has plagued mankind for centuries. Its characteristic flare-ups of intense pain, swelling, and inflammation can disrupt daily life, hinder mobility, and reduce overall well-being. While medications have their place in the treatment of gout, this book delves into the world of natural remedies that can be found right in your kitchen and beyond.

Chapter by chapter, we explore the multifaceted aspects of gout, from understanding its causes and triggers to making lifestyle changes that can make all the difference. We'll begin by delving into the basics of gout, shedding light on its prevalence, risk factors, and the telltale symptoms that accompany its presence. Armed with this knowledge, you will gain a deeper understanding of your condition and the factors that contribute to its development.

We then dive into the pros and cons of commonly prescribed gout medications and provide you with information so you can make informed decisions about your treatment options. While medications can provide relief, we believe that integrating natural remedies into your care plan can complement traditional approaches and improve your overall quality of life.

Diet and lifestyle changes play a key role in the treatment of gout, and in the following chapters we explore the connection between the foods we eat, our lifestyle habits and gout attacks. Find out which foods can trigger gout and learn practical tips for adopting a gout-friendly diet that minimizes the risk of flare-ups. We'll also dive into the power of hydration and explore the benefits of drinking water in flushing out uric acid.

Anti-inflammatory foods are key allies in the fight against gout, and we devote an entire chapter to exploring these nutritional powerhouses. From delicious recipes to ideas for meals rich in anti-inflammatory ingredients, we offer practical advice on how to incorporate these foods into a balanced diet.

But our journey does not end there. We explore the potential benefits of alkaline foods for balancing pH levels, delve into the role of exercise in treating gout, and uncover the healing properties of herbal remedies, essential oils, and homeopathy. The book also explores the potential of common kitchen ingredients such as apple cider vinegar, cherry juice, turmeric, ginger, Epsom salt and baking soda in providing gout relief.

To help you navigate the vast amount of information and options presented, we provide safety precautions, usage guidelines, and recommendations for incorporating these remedies into your daily routine. We also emphasize the importance of long-term lifestyle changes for lasting gout management, including stress management, healthy weight management, and strategies to improve sleep quality.

Through this comprehensive guide, we aim to empower you to take control of your gout and improve your quality of life. By understanding the complexities of this condition and harnessing the power of natural remedies, you can find relief and take a proactive approach to treating gout. Whether you're looking for alternatives to traditional medicine or looking to supplement your existing treatment plan, this book will equip you with the knowledge and tools you need to make informed decisions and restore your vitality.

Join us on this transformational journey as we explore kitchen tools, the power of nature and the path to gout relief. Let's discover the enormous potential that lies within your reach. Together, we can navigate the complexities of the day, strengthen ourselves, and pave the way to a healthier, pain-free future!

Chapter 1:

Understanding Gout: Causes, Symptoms, and Triggers:

Welcome to Chapter 1 of "The Complete Guide to Home Remedies for Gout: From the Kitchen to the Cure." In this chapter, we will embark on a journey of understanding the complexities of gout, a form of arthritis that affects millions of people worldwide. By examining its prevalence, causes, symptoms and triggers, we will lay a solid foundation for effective treatment and relief. So let's delve into the world of days, demystify its complexity and equip ourselves with the knowledge needed to manage this condition.

Overview of gout and its prevalence:

Gout is a type of arthritis characterized by recurring bouts of severe pain, tenderness, redness, and swelling in the joints. It is caused by the accumulation of uric acid crystals in the joints, resulting in inflammation and intense discomfort. Gout most commonly affects the big toe joints, but it can also affect other joints such as the ankles, knees, wrists and fingers.

Gout has been known for centuries, often associated with a lifestyle of excess and indulgence. However, it is important to dispel the myth that gout only affects those who overindulge in rich food and alcohol. While diet can contribute to the development of gout, there are various factors at play that make it a more complex condition than it first appears.

Causes and risk factors for developing gout:

To fully understand gout, we need to examine its underlying causes and the risk factors that contribute to its development. The primary cause of gout is an elevated level of uric acid in the blood, a condition known as hyperuricemia. Uric acid is a by-product of the metabolism of purines, a substance found naturally in the body and in some foods.

Several risk factors increase the likelihood of developing gout. These include:

1 Genetics: Family history and genetics play a role in susceptibility to gout. Some individuals may have a genetic predisposition that makes them more susceptible to developing the condition.

2 Diet: Although diet is not the only cause of gout, certain foods can trigger gout. Foods high in purines, such as red meat, organ meats, seafood, and sugary drinks, can raise uric acid levels and contribute to the development of gout.

3 Obesity: Being overweight puts additional stress on the joints and can lead to increased production of uric acid. Obesity is also related to insulin resistance, which affects uric acid excretion.

4 Medical conditions: Certain medical conditions such as hypertension, diabetes, metabolic syndrome and kidney disease can increase the risk of developing gout.

5 Medications: Certain medications, such as diuretics used to treat hypertension, can interfere with uric acid excretion and contribute to the development of gout.

Common symptoms and signs of gout:

Recognizing the symptoms and signs of gout is essential for prompt diagnosis and effective treatment. The hallmark of gout is an acute gout attack, also known as a flare. Symptoms of a gout attack often develop quickly and peak within 24-48 hours. Common signs and symptoms include:

1. Severe joint pain: Gout attacks are characterized by excruciating pain in the affected joint(s). The pain is often described as throbbing, intense and debilitating.

2. Swelling and redness: The affected joint(s) may swell, be tender to the touch and show noticeable redness.

3. Limited range of motion: During a gout attack, motion of the affected joint(s) may be limited due to pain and swelling, resulting in reduced range of motion.

4. Heat and Warmth: The affected joint(s) may be warm to the touch and the surrounding area may show increased temperature compared to unaffected joints.

5. Recurrent flare-ups: Gout is characterized by recurrent episodes of flare-ups. After the initial attack, symptoms may subside only to reappear later. The frequency and severity of flare-ups can vary from person to person.

Identifying triggers that can lead to gout attacks:

Understanding the triggers that can lead to gout flare-ups is essential to managing and preventing future episodes. While triggers may vary among individuals, some common factors have been identified:

Diet: Certain foods high in purines, such as red meat, organ meats, shellfish and sugary drinks, have been linked to gout flare-ups. Alcohol, especially beer, is also known to trigger gout attacks.

Dehydration: Inadequate hydration can contribute to higher levels of uric acid in the blood, increasing the risk of gout flare-ups. It is important to maintain proper hydration by drinking plenty of water throughout the day.

Medications: Certain medications, such as diuretics and aspirin, can interfere with uric acid excretion and trigger gout flare-ups. It is essential to discuss any medication problems with a healthcare professional.

Injury or trauma: Injury or trauma to the joints can trigger a gout attack in susceptible individuals. It is important to take precautions and practice proper joint protection to minimize the risk of flare-ups.

Stress and illness: High levels of stress and certain illnesses, such as infections or operations, can increase the likelihood of gout flare-ups. Managing stress and taking care of your overall health can help reduce your risk.

By identifying and understanding these triggers, individuals with gout can take proactive steps to minimize exposure and reduce the frequency and severity of gout flares.

Conclusion:

In Chapter 1, we explored the basics of gout, including its prevalence, causes, symptoms, and triggers. Gout is a complex condition influenced by a variety of factors, including genetics, diet, obesity, medical conditions, and medications. Recognizing the symptoms and signs of gout is essential for prompt diagnosis and effective treatment. In addition, identifying triggers that can lead to gout flare-ups allows individuals to make lifestyle changes and take preventative measures.

Armed with this knowledge, we are now ready to delve deeper into the world of gout treatment and explore both conventional and natural remedies. In the following chapters, we will reveal the role of medications, diet and lifestyle changes, anti-inflammatory foods, hydration, exercise, herbal remedies, essential oils, homeopathy, and kitchen remedies. By combining these approaches, we can pave the way to a healthier, pain-free future, taking control of our gout and improving our overall well-being.

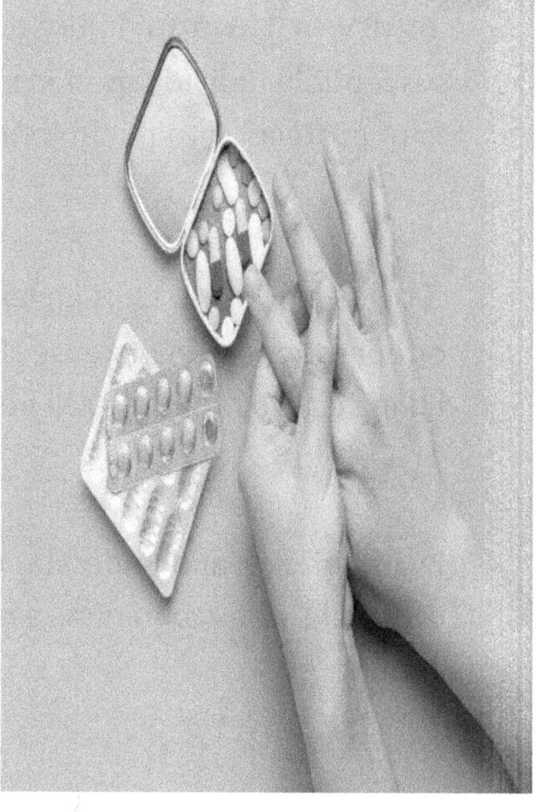

Chapter 2:

Gout Medications: Pros and Cons

When treating gout, medications are often prescribed to relieve symptoms, reduce inflammation, and prevent future gout attacks. This chapter aims to provide an in-depth understanding of commonly prescribed gout medications, their pros and cons, and their essential role in treating the condition. While natural remedies and lifestyle changes are valuable additions to a treatment plan, medications offer targeted relief and support for individuals living with gout.

Overview of commonly prescribed gout medications

The main classes of drugs used to treat gout include nonsteroidal anti-inflammatory drugs (NSAIDs), colchicine, corticosteroids, and xanthine oxidase inhibitors such as allopurinol and febuxostat. NSAIDs such as indomethacin and naproxen are often used to reduce pain and inflammation during acute gout attacks. Colchicine works by inhibiting the inflammatory response and is used both for acute attacks and for prevention. Corticosteroids such as prednisone can be given orally or injected into the affected joint to provide quick relief. Xanthine oxidase inhibitors help reduce the production of uric acid and are used for long-term treatment to prevent gout attacks.

Advantages and disadvantages of gout medications

Gout medications offer several benefits in managing the condition. NSAIDs provide effective pain relief and reduce inflammation, allowing individuals to resume their normal activities. Colchicine can relieve symptoms during acute attacks and can also be used in lower doses for long-term prevention. Corticosteroids provide rapid and powerful anti-inflammatory effects and offer relief from severe gout symptoms. Xanthine oxidase inhibitors help lower uric acid levels over time, reducing the frequency and intensity of gout attacks.

However, gout medications also have potential drawbacks. NSAIDs can cause gastrointestinal side effects, such as stomach pain or ulcers, and may be contraindicated in individuals with kidney problems or those taking blood thinners. Colchicine can cause gastrointestinal symptoms such as diarrhea, especially at higher doses. Corticosteroids, when used for a long time or in high doses, can have systemic side effects such as weight gain, mood changes, and increased blood sugar. Xanthine oxidase inhibitors may cause allergic reactions and may interact with other medications, requiring careful monitoring.

Understanding the role of drugs in the treatment of gout

Medications play a key role in the treatment of gout by providing symptomatic relief during acute attacks, reducing inflammation, and preventing future gout attacks. NSAIDs and colchicine are particularly effective in providing relief during acute attacks, helping individuals regain mobility and reducing pain. Corticosteroids offer rapid relief in severe attacks and may be particularly beneficial when NSAIDs or colchicine are contraindicated or ineffective. Xanthine oxidase inhibitors work by reducing uric acid production and gradually lowering uric acid levels, which helps prevent the formation of urate crystals and subsequent gout attacks.

Discussion of potential side effects and interactions

It is essential to be aware of the potential side effects and interactions associated with gout medications. NSAIDs can cause stomach irritation, ulcers, and an increased risk of cardiovascular events in some individuals. Colchicine can lead to gastrointestinal symptoms such as nausea, vomiting, and diarrhea, especially at higher doses. Corticosteroids, especially when used long-term or in high doses, can have systemic side effects and can interact with other medications. Xanthine oxidase inhibitors may cause skin rashes, liver function abnormalities, and hypersensitivity reactions.

Before starting any gout medication, it is important to consult with a healthcare professional to discuss potential side effects and interactions based on your specific medical history and current medications. They will assess the risks and benefits, taking into account any underlying conditions or contraindications.

Your healthcare provider will carefully monitor your response to the medication and may adjust the dosage or switch to alternative options if necessary. It is important to report any side effects or concerns to your healthcare provider immediately to ensure appropriate treatment and minimize any potential risks.

Adapting the choice of drugs for the treatment of gout

Personalization is key when it comes to choosing the most appropriate gout medication. Factors such as your individual characteristics, medical history, co-existing medical conditions and medication tolerance should be taken into account.

Your healthcare provider will assess your specific needs and adjust your medication selection accordingly. For example, individuals with kidney damage may require medication dosage adjustments or alternative options to minimize the risk of further kidney damage. Similarly, those with a history of gastrointestinal problems may be prescribed drugs that are less likely to cause stomach irritation.

Open communication with your healthcare provider is essential to personalize your medication choices. Be sure to share any concerns, allergies, or adverse reactions you may have experienced in the past to ensure that the medications you are prescribed are the most appropriate for your individual needs.

Conclusion:

Medications are valuable tools in the treatment of gout, providing targeted relief, reducing inflammation, and preventing future gout attacks. However, it is essential to be aware of the advantages and disadvantages associated with these drugs. Understanding their role in gout treatment, as well as potential side effects and interactions, will allow you to make informed decisions about your treatment plan.

Working with your healthcare provider is essential to ensure that medications are tailored to your specific needs, taking into account factors such as your medical history, co-existing conditions, and medication tolerance. By working together, you can optimize your gout treatment and minimize any potential risks associated with medication use. In the following chapters, we'll explore other strategies, including natural remedies and lifestyle changes, to complement your medications and improve your overall gout treatment plan.

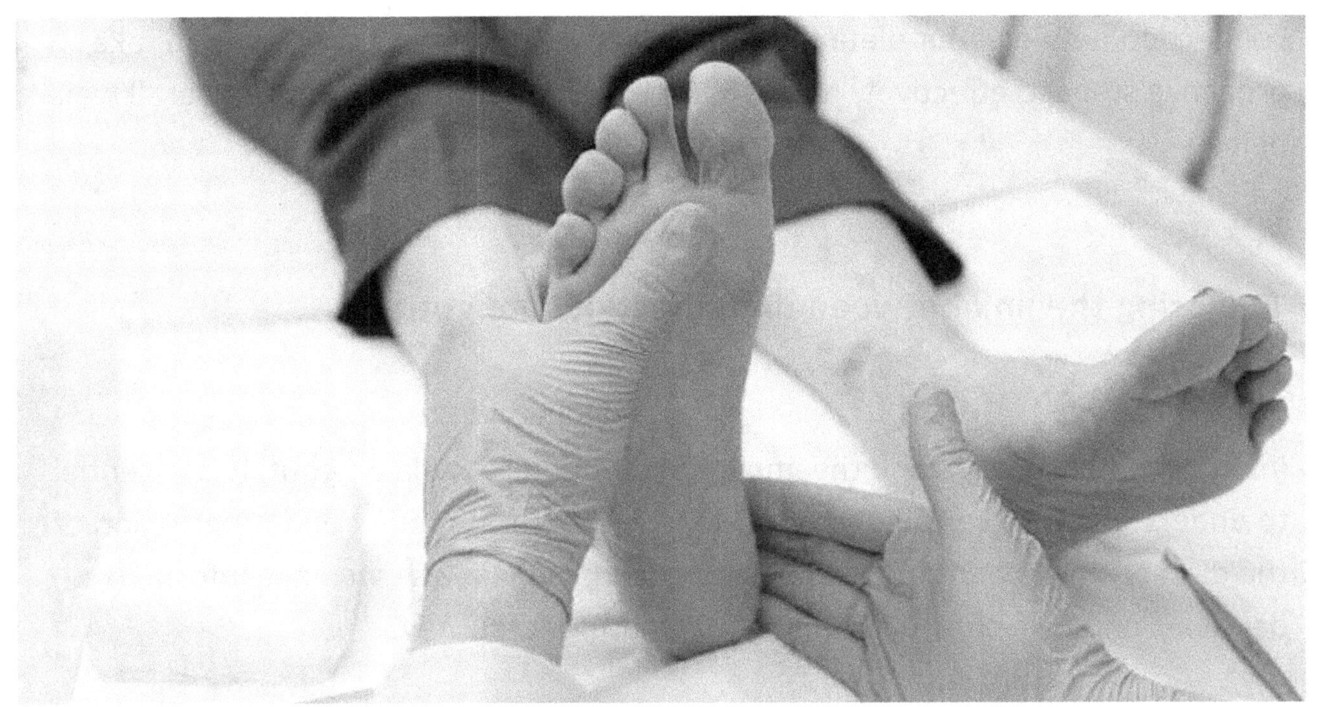

Chapter 3:

Diet and Lifestyle Changes for Gout Management

In this chapter, we will explore the profound impact of diet and lifestyle on treating gout. While medications play a role in relieving gout symptoms, adopting a gout-friendly diet and making positive lifestyle changes can significantly reduce the frequency and severity of gout attacks. By understanding the complex connection between our dietary choices, lifestyle habits and gout, we can take proactive steps to effectively manage the condition and improve our overall well-being.

Exploring the link between diet, lifestyle and gout

In order to fully understand the impact of diet and lifestyle on gout, it is essential to understand how certain factors influence the development and progression of the disease. By recognizing these connections, individuals can make informed decisions and take control of their gout treatment journey.

One critical aspect to consider is the role of purines in gout. Purines are natural compounds found in various foods that break down into uric acid when consumed. Excessive levels of uric acid can lead to the formation of urate crystals that trigger painful gout flare-ups. By understanding which foods are high in purines, individuals can make choices to minimize their impact on uric acid levels and gout symptoms.

Identifying foods that can trigger gout attacks

Certain foods are known to be potential triggers for gout flare-ups due to their high purine content. These include organ meats such as liver and kidney, seafood such as anchovies and sardines, and some vegetables such as mushrooms and asparagus. By knowing these high-purine foods, individuals can adjust their eating habits to reduce the risk of gout flare-ups.

In addition to avoiding foods high in purines, moderation and portion control are essential. Some foods have moderate levels of purines and can still be enjoyed in moderation without significantly increasing uric acid levels. By practicing portion control and being mindful of total purine intake, individuals can achieve a balance between their dietary preferences and gout treatment goals.

However, it's not all about limitations. Certain foods have potential benefits for treating gout. For example, low-fat dairy products are associated with a reduced risk of gout flare-ups. Naturally low in purines, fruits and vegetables provide essential nutrients and can be incorporated into a gout-friendly diet to support overall health.

Tips for Adopting a Gout-Friendly Diet

Adopting a gout-friendly diet goes beyond avoiding trigger foods. It involves adopting a balanced and varied diet that promotes overall well-being while minimizing the risk of gout attacks.

A key component of a gout-friendly diet is focusing on fiber-rich foods. Foods high in fiber, such as whole grains, legumes, and certain vegetables, can promote healthy digestion and potentially help lower uric acid levels. By incorporating these foods into meals and snacks, individuals can promote optimal gut health and potentially alleviate gout symptoms.

Limiting alcohol consumption is another crucial aspect of a gout-friendly diet. Alcohol, especially beer and spirits, can significantly increase the risk of gout attacks. Individuals with gout are advised to limit their alcohol intake, or in some cases avoid it altogether, to minimize the impact on uric acid levels and gout symptoms.

Incorporating healthy lifestyle habits to treat gout

Maintaining a healthy weight is of utmost importance. Being overweight further puts stress on the joints, including those affected by gout. By eating a balanced diet rich in whole foods and low in processed foods and sugary drinks, individuals can achieve and maintain a healthy weight. Regular physical activity is also essential in managing gout. Joint-friendly exercise, such as swimming or cycling, can help strengthen muscles, improve joint mobility and reduce the frequency of gout attacks.

Managing comorbidities is another important aspect of gout management. Gout often coexists with other medical conditions such as hypertension and diabetes. By effectively managing these comorbidities through lifestyle changes and appropriate medical interventions, individuals can improve their overall health and potentially reduce the incidence of gout.

Stress management and sleep quality should not be overlooked when treating gout. High levels of stress and lack of sleep can trigger gout attacks. It is essential to develop effective stress management techniques such as relaxation exercises, meditation or engaging in hobbies that bring joy and relaxation. In addition, prioritizing quality sleep by establishing a regular sleep schedule and creating a comfortable sleep environment can help reduce gout symptoms.

Conclusion:

By understanding the complex relationship between diet, lifestyle and gout, individuals can take charge of their gout healing journey. Adopting a gout-friendly diet that emphasizes low-purine foods, portion control, and a balanced diet can help reduce the risk of gout flare-ups. Incorporating healthy lifestyle habits, including maintaining a healthy weight, managing comorbidities, and practicing stress management techniques can further support gout management efforts.

Remember that each individual's experience with gout may vary and it is essential to work closely with healthcare professionals to tailor dietary and lifestyle recommendations to specific needs. By making an informed decision, individuals can proactively manage gout, reduce the frequency and severity of flare-ups, and improve their overall quality of life.

Chapter 4:

The Best Anti-Inflammatory Foods for Gout Relief

In this chapter, we explore the remarkable power of anti-inflammatory foods in providing gout relief. Gout is characterized by chronic inflammation that leads to painful flare-ups and joint damage. By incorporating specific foods with strong anti-inflammatory properties into your diet, you can significantly reduce inflammation, manage gout symptoms, and promote overall joint health.

Understanding the power of anti-inflammatory foods

Overview of anti-inflammatory foods:

Chronic inflammation lies at the heart of gout, contributing to its painful symptoms and long-term complications. This section provides a comprehensive understanding of inflammation and its role in gout. Introducing the concept of anti-inflammatory foods that are rich in compounds that fight inflammation. By adopting an anti-inflammatory diet, you can harness the healing power of these foods to reduce the inflammation associated with gout.

Exploring the benefits:

In this section, we will delve into the many benefits of anti-inflammatory foods for people with gout. We discuss how these foods work to reduce inflammation and relieve symptoms such as joint pain, swelling, and redness. By incorporating these foods into your daily routine, you can experience long-term effects that go beyond gout relief, including improved overall health and reduced risk of chronic disease.

Specific foods for gout relief

Berry:

Berries such as strawberries, blueberries, raspberries and cherries are bursting with antioxidants and anti-inflammatory compounds. We explore the unique benefits of each type of berry and how they can help reduce the inflammation associated with gout. In addition to their benefits, we provide practical tips on how to incorporate these tasty fruits into your meals, snacks and smoothies to increase their anti-inflammatory properties.

Green leafy vegetables:

Green leafy vegetables, including spinach, kale, chard and leafy greens, are a source of nutrients that have exceptional anti-inflammatory properties. We highlight the nutritional value and unique benefits of each green and discuss how they can help reduce gout inflammation. In addition, we provide a variety of recipes and meal ideas that creatively incorporate leafy greens to make them a delicious and integral part of your diet.

Foods rich in omega-3 fatty acids:

Omega-3 fatty acids are widely recognized for their anti-inflammatory effects. We are researching a variety of omega-3 sources, including fatty fish (salmon, mackerel, sardines), walnuts, flaxseeds, and chia seeds. By incorporating these foods into your diet, you can harness the power of omega-3s to reduce inflammation and relieve gout symptoms. We provide practical suggestions and easy-to-understand tips for adding these omega-3 rich foods to your daily meals.

Turmeric:

Turmeric contains a powerful anti-inflammatory compound called curcumin, which has been extensively studied for its therapeutic effects. Let's dive into the remarkable anti-inflammatory benefits of turmeric and curcumin in treating gout symptoms. In addition, we provide practical guidelines for incorporating turmeric into a variety of recipes, including curries, smoothies, teas and golden milk, to maximize its effectiveness.

Ginger:

Ginger has a long-standing reputation for its anti-inflammatory and analgesic properties. In this section, we explore the unique benefits of ginger in reducing gout-related inflammation. We discuss different ways to incorporate ginger into your diet, including using it in teas, smoothies, stir-fries and dressings. Explore the diverse culinary possibilities of this **powerful anti-inflammatory root with our recipes and meal ideas.**

Recipes and meal ideas

Berry Blast Smoothie:

Recipe:

Ingredients:

1 cup mixed fruit (strawberries, blueberries, raspberries)

1 ripe banana

1 cup unsweetened almond milk or Greek yogurt

1 tablespoon of chia seeds

1 tablespoon honey or maple syrup (optional for extra sweetness)

Ice cubes (optional)

Instruction:

Wash the fruit thoroughly and remove any stems or leaves.

Peel and slice the banana.

In a blender, combine the blended berries, banana, almond milk or Greek yogurt, chia seeds, and sweetener (if desired).

Blend on high speed until smooth and creamy.

If you like, add a few ice cubes and blend again for a chilled and refreshing texture.

Pour the smoothie into a glass and serve immediately.

Variation:

For added protein, add a scoop of protein powder or a tablespoon of almond butter to your smoothie.

To increase the nutritional content, add a handful of spinach or kale to the blender and create a green berry smoothie.

Adjust the sweetness by adjusting the amount of honey or maple syrup to suit your taste preferences.

Experiment with different combinations of berries or add a splash of citrus juice for a zesty twist.

Mediterranean Salad:

Recipe:

Ingredients:

2 cups mixed salad greens (spinach, arugula, romaine)

1 medium cucumber, diced

1 cup cherry tomatoes, halved

1/2 red onion, thinly sliced

1/4 cup Kalamata olives, pitted

1/4 cup crumbled feta cheese

2 tablespoons of extra virgin olive oil

1 tablespoon of lemon juice

1 teaspoon of dried oregano

Salt and pepper to taste

Instruction:

In a large salad bowl, combine the mixed lettuce, cucumber, cherry tomatoes, red onion, Kalamata olives and feta cheese.

In a separate small bowl, whisk together the olive oil, lemon juice, dried oregano, salt and pepper to make the dressing.

Pour the dressing over the salad and toss gently to coat all the ingredients.

Let the flavors meld for a few minutes before serving.

Serve the Mediterranean salad as a light and refreshing main course or as a side dish.

Variation:

Add grilled chicken or shrimp for a heartier meal.

Add chopped peppers, artichoke hearts, or roasted red peppers for extra flavor and texture.

For a vegan version, omit the feta cheese or substitute vegan cheese or tofu.

Customize the dressing by adding balsamic vinegar or Dijon mustard for a tangy flavor.

Turmeric Ginger Golden Milk:

Recipe:

Ingredients:

1 cup unsweetened almond milk or coconut milk

1 teaspoon ground turmeric

1/2 teaspoon ground ginger

1/2 teaspoon cinnamon

1 tablespoon of honey or maple syrup

A pinch of black pepper (optional)

pinch of vanilla extract (optional)

Instruction:

In a small saucepan, heat the almond milk or coconut milk over medium heat until warm but not boiling.

Add ground turmeric, ground ginger, cinnamon, honey or maple syrup, black pepper (if using), and vanilla extract (if using).

Whisk the ingredients until well combined and the mixture is smooth.

Continue heating the golden milk mixture, stirring occasionally, until it reaches the desired temperature.

Remove from heat and pour the golden milk into a mug.

Enjoy the turmeric-ginger golden milk warm and enjoy

Chapter 5:

Benefits of drinking water for gout

In the field of gout treatment, there are few remedies as simple yet effective as water. This chapter delves into the vital role of hydration in the treatment of gout and examines how water can effectively help flush out uric acid, a key contributor to gout attacks. By understanding the importance of staying adequately hydrated and exploring other hydration drinks, you can take significant steps toward managing gout symptoms and promoting overall well-being.

The importance of hydration in the treatment of gout

Understanding the connection between hydration and gout:

Proper hydration is vital to overall health and plays a key role in treating gout. When you are well hydrated, it helps dilute the concentration of uric acid in your blood, making it easier for your body to eliminate excess uric acid through urine. Conversely, insufficient hydration can lead to higher levels of uric acid, increasing the risk of gout flare-ups. Understanding this connection highlights the importance of hydration as an essential element in the treatment of gout.

Benefits of adequate hydration:

Adequate hydration offers numerous benefits for treating gout. By keeping your body well hydrated, you can help reduce the concentration of uric acid in your joints and minimize the formation of uric acid crystals, reducing the likelihood of painful gout flare-ups. In addition, proper hydration supports efficient kidney function and allows the kidneys to effectively filter and excrete uric acid. This in turn helps prevent gout attacks and contributes to overall kidney health.

Water: Your perfect hydration ally

Understanding the role of water in flushing out uric acid:

Water plays a vital role in dissolving and excreting uric acid from the body. When you consume enough water, it helps dilute the uric acid present in your blood and joints, making it easier for your body to excrete it through urine. The hydration provided by water also supports optimal kidney function, facilitating the filtration of waste products including uric acid. By ensuring proper hydration through water consumption, you are actively helping your body to effectively eliminate uric acid, thereby reducing the risk of gout attacks.

Tips for staying adequately hydrated:

To reap the benefits of hydration for gout treatment, it is essential to stay consistently and adequately hydrated. Here are some practical tips to help you achieve optimal hydration levels:

- **Set optimal daily water intake goals:** While the exact amount of water needed can vary based on factors such as age, weight, and activity level, a general recommendation is to aim for at least 8 cups (64 ounces) of water per day.

However, individuals with gout may require a higher water intake to increase uric acid excretion.

- **Spread your water consumption throughout the day:** Drink water consistently throughout the day, rather than consuming large amounts at once. This ensures a constant supply of hydration and supports optimal body functions.

- **Set reminders and build habits:** Use reminders such as alarms or smartphone apps to encourage yourself to drink water regularly. You can also create habits like drinking a glass of water when you wake up or before a meal to incorporate hydration into your daily routine.

- **Keep water accessible:** Carry a reusable water bottle with you wherever you go. Having water readily available makes it easier to stay hydrated, especially when you're on the go or in situations where access to water may be limited.

Exploring other hydration drinks and their effect on gout

Herbal teas and infusions:

In addition to water, herbal teas and infusions can contribute to your hydration goals while offering other health benefits. Certain herbal teas, such as chamomile, ginger, and green tea, have anti-inflammatory properties that can help reduce gout inflammation. They also provide a tasty alternative to plain water. Experiment with different herbal teas to find ones you like and that work with your gout treatment plan.

Fruit and vegetable juices:

Fruit and vegetable juices can provide hydration along with essential nutrients and antioxidants. Opt for freshly squeezed juices or those without added sugar or preservatives. Certain fruits and vegetables, such as cherries and celery, have been shown to have anti-inflammatory properties that can help relieve gout symptoms. Include these juices in your diet to enjoy their hydrating benefits while supporting your overall gout treatment plan.

Electrolyte enhanced drinks:

Drinks high in electrolytes, such as coconut water and sports drinks, can be helpful for replenishing electrolytes and staying hydrated, especially during periods of vigorous physical activity or sweating. However, pay attention to their sugar content and choose variants with a minimum of added sugars. These drinks can help with hydration and electrolyte balance, which can indirectly support gout treatment by promoting overall health and well-being.

Restrictions on dehydrating drinks:

While we're focusing on hydration drinks, it's equally important to know about drinks that can contribute to dehydration and potentially trigger gout. Alcoholic drinks, sugary drinks and caffeinated drinks have diuretic effects, which can increase urine production and lead to dehydration. Limit your intake of these beverages or avoid them altogether to maintain proper hydration levels and minimize the risk of gout flare-ups.

Conclusion:

In conclusion, water serves as the ultimate hydration ally in the treatment of gout. It plays a vital role in flushing out uric acid, reducing the risk of gout flare-ups and supporting overall kidney health. By staying well-hydrated, you will help your body eliminate uric acid effectively. In addition, exploring other hydration beverages such as herbal teas, fruit and vegetable juices, and electrolyte drinks can provide variety and additional health benefits. Remember to limit or avoid dehydrating drinks, which can worsen gout symptoms. By making hydration a fundamental aspect of your gout treatment plan, you will empower yourself to take control of your health and promote overall well-being.

Chapter 6:

Alkaline foods to balance pH levels and reduce gout attacks

In this chapter, we delve into the interesting concept of alkaline foods and their potential role in balancing pH levels and reducing gout flare-ups. Gout, often associated with high levels of uric acid in the blood, can be affected by the body's pH balance. By understanding the relationship between pH levels and gout, we can explore how incorporating alkaline foods into our diet can help manage the condition and promote overall well-being.

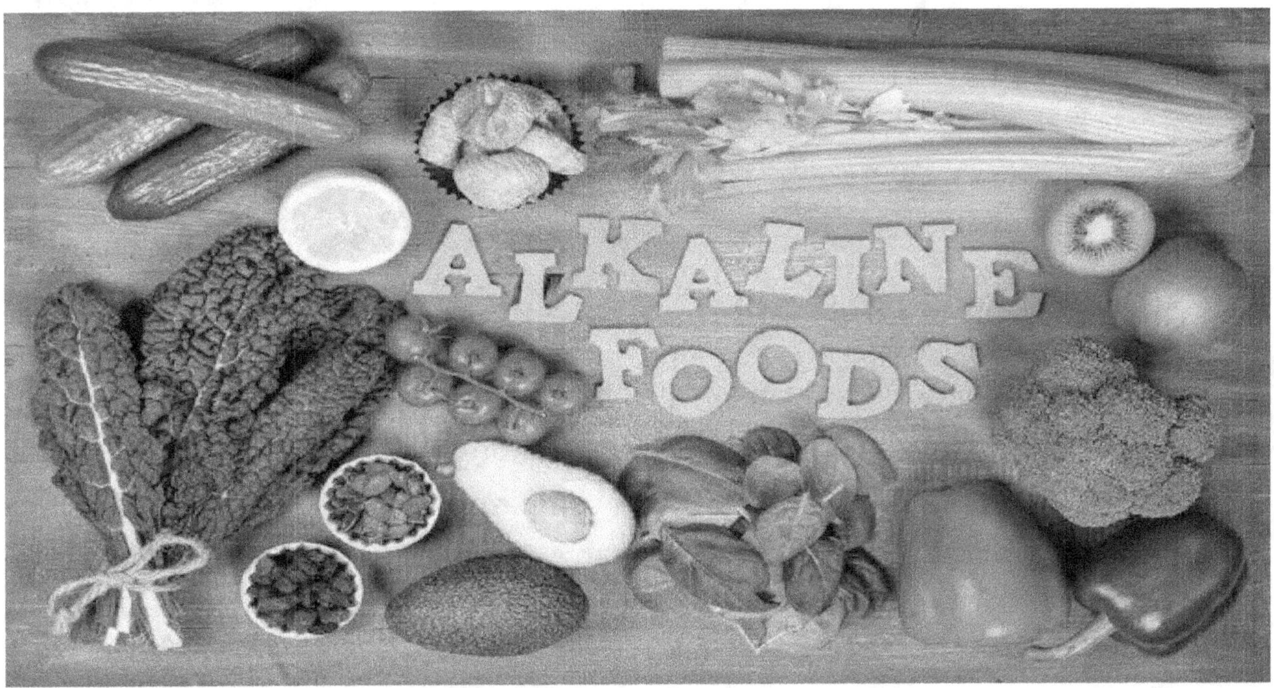

Relationship between pH levels and gout:

To understand the effect of alkaline foods on gout, it is essential to understand the relationship between pH levels and the body's internal environment. pH is a measure of acidity or alkalinity and is shown on a scale of 0 to 14, with 7 being neutral. The body naturally maintains a slightly alkaline pH, around 7.35 to 7.45, to support optimal physiological functions.

Gout is associated with high levels of uric acid, a byproduct of purine metabolism. When uric acid crystallizes and builds up in the joints, it triggers inflammation and excruciating pain. Studies suggest that an acidic environment can facilitate the formation of uric acid crystals, which worsen gout symptoms. By promoting an alkaline environment, we can potentially counteract this process and alleviate gout symptoms.

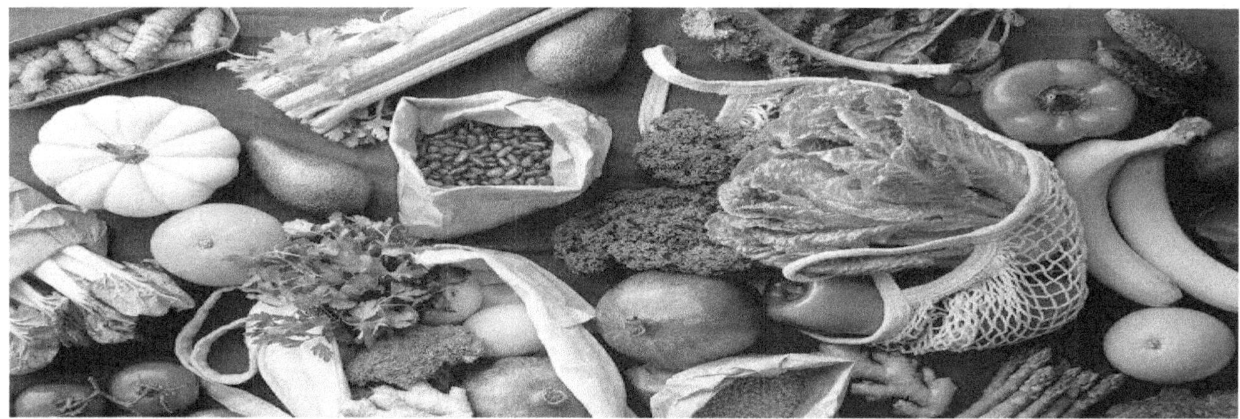

Identifying alkaline foods and their potential benefits:

Alkaline foods are those that have an alkalizing effect on the body when metabolized. They help balance acidity and promote a more alkaline pH. While the body maintains its pH balance through complex physiological mechanisms, incorporating alkaline foods into our diet can support these processes and reduce the risk of gout flare-ups.

Some examples of alkaline foods include fresh fruits and vegetables such as leafy greens, cucumbers, avocados, broccoli, and citrus fruits. These foods are rich in minerals and have an alkalizing effect on the body when consumed. Additionally, certain nuts, seeds and whole grains such as almonds, quinoa and millet can also contribute to a more alkaline pH.

Potential benefits of alkaline foods for treating gout include reducing inflammation, promoting joint health, and promoting overall well-being. By incorporating these nutrient-dense foods into our meals, we provide our bodies with essential vitamins, minerals and antioxidants that contribute to a balanced internal environment.

Recipes and meal suggestions with alkaline-rich ingredients:

To help you incorporate alkaline foods into your daily meals, we've provided a selection of recipes and meal ideas that showcase these pH-balancing ingredients. The goal of these recipes is not only to relieve the symptoms of gout, but also to tantalize your taste buds and make healthy eating a pleasant experience.

1. Alkaline Green Smoothie: Blend spinach, cucumber, celery, lime juice and a handful of parsley for a refreshing and alkalizing green smoothie. Packed with alkali-rich vegetables, this vibrant drink is an excellent choice for a gout-friendly breakfast or snack.

2. Grilled salmon with lemon and dill: Marinate fresh salmon fillets in lemon juice, dill and a little olive oil, then grill to perfection. This dish combines alkaline lemon juice with omega-3 fatty acids from salmon to provide a nutritious and delicious option for lunch or dinner.

3. Quinoa Salad with Mixed Greens: Combine cooked quinoa with a mix of alkaline vegetables like cherry tomatoes, peppers, cucumbers and fresh herbs.

Drizzle with lemon vinaigrette for a tangy and tangy salad that can be enjoyed as a main course or side dish.

4. Almond and Berry Parfait: Layer unsweetened almond yogurt with a variety of tart berries like blueberries, raspberries, and strawberries. Top with toasted almonds for extra crunch and enjoy this alkali-rich dessert or snack.

5. Roasted Vegetable Mix: Toss basic vegetables like zucchini, eggplant, peppers and onions with olive oil, garlic and herbs. Roast them in the oven until soft and caramelized. This tasty and nutrient-dense dish can be served as a hearty side dish or as a vegetarian main course.

6. Citrus Water: Pour your water with alkaline citrus fruits like lemons, limes and oranges. Simply cut up the fruit and add it to a pitcher of water. Let the flavors meld overnight in the fridge and enjoy this refreshing and hydrating drink throughout the day.

These are just a few examples of recipes and meal ideas that contain alkaline-rich ingredients. By incorporating these alkaline foods into your meals, you can create a gout-friendly diet that will not only support your overall health, but also help manage your gout symptoms.

In conclusion, incorporating alkaline foods into your diet has the potential to balance pH levels, reduce inflammation, and alleviate gout flare-ups. When you understand the relationship between pH levels and gout, you can make informed choices about the foods you eat. With recipes and meal suggestions provided, you can explore the world of alkaline-rich ingredients and embark on a culinary journey that supports your gout goals. Remember, nourishing your body with alkaline foods is a step toward finding relief and achieving a healthier, pain-free life.

Chapter 7:

The role of exercise in the treatment of gout

Welcome to Chapter 7 of "The Complete Guide to Home Remedies for Gout: From the Kitchen to the Cure." In this chapter, we will explore the important role that exercise plays in the treatment of gout. While it may seem counterintuitive to engage in physical activity when experiencing gout symptoms, exercise can actually be a powerful tool for relieving pain, reducing inflammation, and preventing future gout flare-ups. In the following pages, we'll delve into the importance of exercise in managing gout, discuss low-impact exercises suitable for individuals with gout, provide tips on how to incorporate regular physical activity into your daily routine, and highlight the many benefits of exercise for both overall health and gout prevention.

Understanding the importance of exercise for treating gout:

Regular exercise is a key part of an effective gout treatment plan. Physical activity contributes to improving blood circulation, strengthening muscles and joints, maintaining a healthy weight and improving overall joint function. By incorporating exercise into your routine, you can help reduce the frequency and severity of gout attacks as well as improve your overall quality of life.

Discussing low-impact exercises suitable for individuals with gout:

When it comes to exercise for gout, it's important to choose activities that are gentle on your joints and minimize the risk of injury or worsening gout symptoms. Low-impact exercises are ideal in this regard. These exercises provide the benefits of physical activity with minimal stress on the joints. Some suitable low-impact exercises for individuals with gout include walking, swimming, cycling, water aerobics, tai chi, and yoga. We'll examine each of these exercises in detail, discuss their benefits, and provide instructions on how to safely incorporate them into your routine.

Tips for incorporating regular physical activity into your daily routine:

Finding the motivation and time to exercise regularly can be challenging, but with the right strategies, it can become an enjoyable and sustainable part of your daily routine. In this section, we bring you practical tips and suggestions on how to include regular physical activity in your busy schedule. From setting achievable goals to finding activities you enjoy and creating a consistent exercise routine, these tips will help you overcome obstacles and maintain long-term adherence to your exercise regimen.

Benefits of exercise for overall health and gout prevention:

The benefits of exercise extend far beyond treating gout. Regular physical activity offers a wide range of benefits for your overall health and well-being. In this section, we delve into the many benefits that exercise provides, including improved cardiovascular health, increased muscle strength and flexibility, improved mood and well-being, weight management, and reduced risk of co-morbidities such as diabetes and heart disease. We're also looking at how exercise can prevent future gout attacks by lowering uric acid levels, promoting healthy weight management and improving overall joint health.

Incorporating exercise into your daily routine can be transformative for your gout treatment and your overall health. By understanding the importance of exercise, discovering low-impact exercises suitable for individuals with gout, implementing practical tips for regular physical activity, and recognizing the comprehensive benefits that exercise offers, you can take proactive steps to effectively manage your gout and improve your quality of life. Let's dive into the world of exercise and unlock its potential for gout relief and overall well-being.

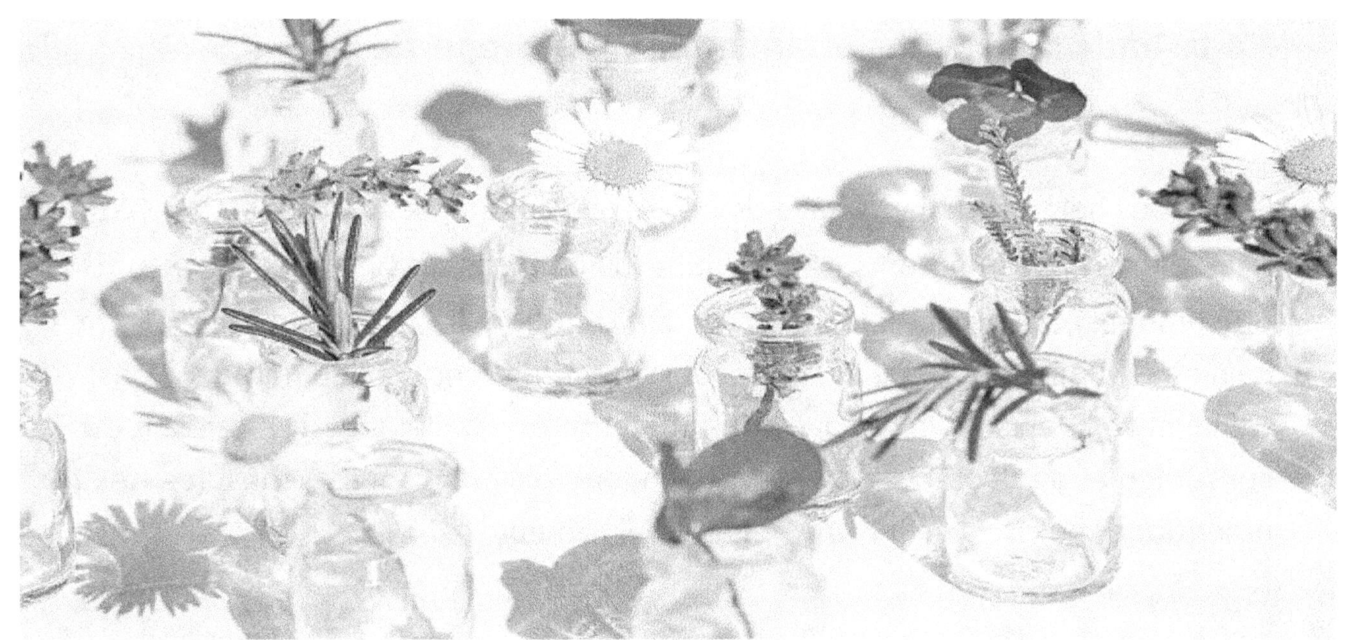

Chapter 8:

Herbal Remedies for Gout: The Healing Power of Nature

Herbal remedies have been used for centuries to alleviate various ailments, and gout is no exception. In this chapter, we delve into the world of herbal gout remedies and explore the power of natural medicinal plants in providing relief from the symptoms of this debilitating condition. Herbal remedies offer a natural and holistic approach to treating gout, using the anti-inflammatory properties of certain herbs and plants to reduce pain and inflammation.

Herbs and plants with anti-inflammatory properties:

Numerous herbs and plants have powerful anti-inflammatory properties that can help relieve gout symptoms. One such herb is **devil's claw** (Harpagophytum procumbens), which has long been used in traditional medicine to relieve joint pain and inflammation. Devil's claw contains compounds called harpagosides, which have been shown to have anti-inflammatory and analgesic effects. It can be consumed as a tea or in supplement form, but it is important to consult a health practitioner before starting any new herbal remedy.

Another herb renowned for its anti-inflammatory properties is **turmeric** (Curcuma longa). The active ingredient in turmeric, curcumin, has been studied extensively for its ability to reduce inflammation. It inhibits various inflammatory pathways in the body and can be consumed as supplements or incorporated into foods and beverages. Combining turmeric with black pepper increases its absorption because black pepper contains a compound called piperine that improves the bioavailability of curcumin.

Boswellia (Boswellia serrata), commonly known as Indian frankincense, is another powerful herb for gout relief. It contains boswellic acids, which exhibit anti-inflammatory and analgesic properties. Boswellia can be taken as a supplement or topically as a cream or ointment to soothe inflamed joints.

Preparation and use of herbal preparations at home:

When it comes to preparing herbal remedies at home, there are various methods that you can explore.

One popular option is **herbal teas**, which can be prepared by infusing herbs in hot water. For gout relief, consider making a tea with herbs such as nettle leaf (Urtica dioica) or ginger (Zingiber officinale), both of which have anti-inflammatory properties. Sipping these teas throughout the day can help reduce inflammation and provide relief.

Another approach is to create **poultices** or poultices from herbs such as chamomile (Matricaria chamomilla) or comfrey (Symphytum officinale). These herbs can be crushed, mixed with warm water or carrier oils and applied directly to the affected joints. The warmth and herbal properties help relieve pain and inflammation.

Precautions and possible drug interactions:

While herbal remedies can be effective for gout relief, it is important to exercise caution and be aware of potential drug interactions. Some herbs can interfere with the absorption or metabolism of certain medications, leading to unintended consequences. Therefore, it is imperative to consult with a healthcare professional or qualified herbalist before incorporating herbal remedies into your gout treatment plan, especially if you are currently taking medication.

In addition, pregnant or breastfeeding women should exercise caution when using herbal preparations, as some herbs may have adverse effects. Always consult a healthcare professional before using any herbal medicine during these periods.

In addition, it is important to source herbs and herbal products from reputable suppliers to ensure quality and safety. If you are harvesting herbs from your garden or in the wild, be sure to properly identify them and research any side effects or contraindications.

Conclusion:

Herbal remedies offer a natural and complementary approach to treating gout, harnessing the power of plants to reduce pain and inflammation. Incorporating herbs such as devil's claw, turmeric, and boswellia into your gout treatment plan can provide additional relief and support the overall well-being of your joints.

However, it is essential to approach herbal medicines with caution and seek advice from health professionals or herbalists. Precautions should be taken, especially if you are currently taking medications, as some herbs may interact with them. Additionally, those who are pregnant or breastfeeding should take extra care and consult with their health care providers before using herbal products.

When making herbal remedies at home, consider brewing herbal teas or creating compresses and poultices using anti-inflammatory herbs such as nettle leaf, ginger, chamomile, or comfrey. These natural treatments can be incorporated into your daily routine to help relieve gout symptoms and promote a sense of well-being.

Be sure to buy herbs and herbal products from reputable suppliers to ensure their quality and safety. If you choose to harvest herbs from your garden or the wild, ensure proper identification and research any side effects or contraindications.

In conclusion, we can say that herbal preparations offer a natural and holistic approach to the treatment of gout, using the healing power of natural plants. By exploring the anti-inflammatory properties of herbs like devil's claw, turmeric, and boswellia and incorporating them into your gout treatment plan, you can increase the relief and support provided by traditional treatments. With proper care, guidance, and knowledge, herbal remedies can be valuable allies on your journey to treating gout and promoting overall joint health. Embrace nature's gifts and discover the potential of herbal medicine in your quest for a pain-free and vibrant life.

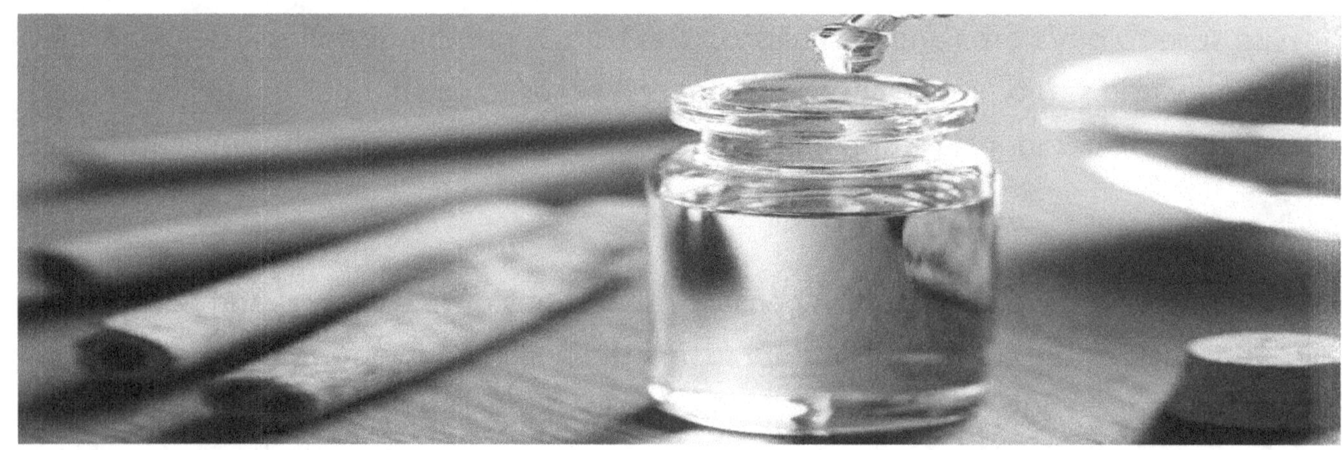

Chapter 9:

Essential Oils for Gout: Aromatherapy for Pain Relief

In this chapter, we delve into the world of essential oils and their potential benefits in reducing the pain and inflammation associated with gout. Essential oils have long been valued for their aromatic properties and therapeutic potential. Their concentrated plant extracts contain compounds known for their anti-inflammatory and analgesic properties, making them a promising natural remedy for gout relief.

Understanding Essential Oils:

Essential oils are highly concentrated liquids derived from various plant sources such as flowers, leaves, bark and roots. These oils capture the essence and fragrance of the plant as well as its healing properties. Each essential oil has a unique composition of bioactive substances that contribute to its therapeutic effects.

Benefits of essential oils for gout:

Essential oils offer a number of benefits for individuals with gout. They have been found to have anti-inflammatory properties, help reduce swelling, and relieve pain associated with gout flare-ups. In addition, some essential oils exhibit analgesic effects and provide natural pain relief. Their aromatic nature also promotes relaxation and can help manage stress, which can be beneficial for those experiencing gout-related discomfort.

Essential Oils for Gout Relief:

Several essential oils have shown potential in treating gout symptoms. Here are some examples:

1. Frankincense Oil: Known for its anti-inflammatory properties, frankincense oil can help reduce the inflammation and pain associated with gout. Its soothing aroma can also provide stress relief.

2. Lavender Oil: Lavender oil is known for its soothing properties. It can help relieve pain, reduce inflammation, and promote relaxation, which helps manage gout symptoms.

3. Peppermint Oil: Peppermint oil contains menthol, a compound known for its cooling and analgesic effects. Topical application of diluted peppermint oil can help relieve pain and provide a refreshing sensation.

4. Rosemary Oil: Rosemary oil has anti-inflammatory properties and can help reduce the inflammation associated with gout. Its stimulating aroma can also energize and promote mental clarity.

Ways to use essential oils for gout relief:

There are different ways to incorporate essential oils into your gout treatment plan. Here are some methods to consider:

1. Topical application: Dilute the essential oil with a carrier oil such as coconut or jojoba oil and apply directly to the affected area. Gently massage the oil into the skin to promote absorption and relief.

2. Aromatherapy: Diffuse essential oils in a diffuser or inhale the aroma directly from the bottle. Aromatherapy can help relax the mind, relieve stress and provide a sense of overall well-being.

3. Compresses: Make a warm or cold compress by adding a few drops of essential oil to a bowl of warm or cold water. Soak a clean cloth in the mixture, wring it out and apply it to the affected area for localized relief.

Safety instructions and instructions for use:

While essential oils can provide natural relief, it is essential to use them safely and responsibly. Here are some guidelines to consider:

1. Dilution: Always dilute essential oils with a suitable carrier oil before applying topically. This helps prevent skin irritation or sensitization. Follow the recommended dilution ratios and test the patch on a small area of skin before wider use.

2. Quality and Purity: Choose high-quality, pure essential oils from reputable sources to ensure their therapeutic efficacy and avoid potential contaminants.

3. Sensitivity and Allergies: Individuals with sensitive skin or known allergies should exercise caution when using essential oils. Do a patch test and discontinue use if adverse reactions occur.

4. Consultation: If you have any underlying medical conditions or are currently taking medication, it is advisable to consult a healthcare professional before using essential oils for gout relief. They can provide you with personalized advice based on your specific circumstances.

5. Air Quality: When using essential oils using diffusers or inhalation methods, ensure proper ventilation to prevent overexposure and maintain air quality.

6. Storage: Store essential oils in dark, airtight bottles away from direct sunlight, heat and moisture to preserve their potency and extend their shelf life.

Conclusion:

Essential oils offer a natural and aromatic approach to treating gout symptoms. Due to their anti-inflammatory and analgesic properties, these concentrated plant extracts can provide relief from the pain and inflammation associated with gout. Whether through topical application, aromatherapy, or compresses, essential oils offer a versatile and enjoyable way to incorporate natural remedies into your gout treatment routine.

However, when working with essential oils, it is important to prioritize safety and proper usage guidelines. Diluting, ensuring quality, considering sensitivities, and seeking professional advice are essential steps to effective use of essential oils.

In the next chapter, we will explore the fascinating world of homeopathy and its potential role in providing relief from gout symptoms. By understanding the principles and remedies of homeopathy, you can further expand your options for holistic and personalized approaches to treating gout.

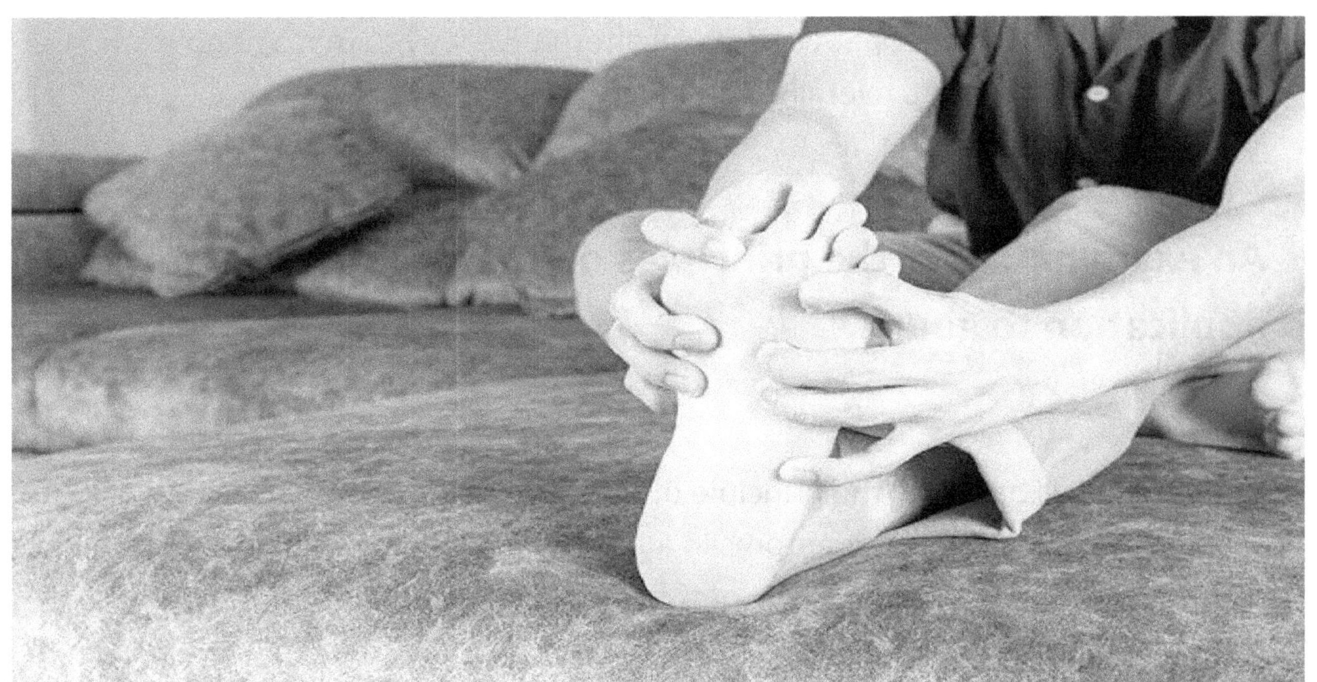

Chapter 10:

Homeopathy for Gout: Treating Symptoms with Natural Remedies

In this chapter we delve into the fascinating field of homeopathy and its application in the treatment of gout. Homeopathy is a holistic healing system that has gained recognition for its gentle yet effective approach to restoring balance and promoting wellness. With its emphasis on individualized treatment and natural remedies, homeopathy offers an alternative way to manage gout symptoms and promote overall well-being.

An examination of the principles of homeopathy and its application to gout:

Homeopathy is based on the principle of "like cures like". This means that a substance that can cause symptoms in a healthy individual can be used in a highly diluted form to treat similar symptoms in a person suffering from the disease. Homeopathic medicines are derived from a variety of substances, including plants, minerals and animals, and are prepared through a careful process of dilution and potentiation.

When it comes to gout, homeopathy aims to address the underlying imbalance and restore harmony in the body. It recognizes the unique nature of each individual and tries to tailor treatment to that, taking into account the person's specific symptoms, triggers and overall health picture.

Discussion of common homeopathic remedies for gout symptoms:

Homeopathic gout remedies target both acute flare-ups and chronic symptoms. Although it is essential to consult a qualified homeopath for personal advice, several commonly used remedies show promise in providing relief. Here are some examples:

1. Colchicum: This medicine is often indicated for gout characterized by intense pain and inflammation that worsens with the slightest touch. Affected joints may be swollen, hot and red, and the pain tends to be worse at night.

2. Ledum palustre: When the symptoms of gout primarily affect smaller joints such as the toes or ankles and there is a feeling of coolness and relief from the application of cold, Ledum palustre may be prescribed. It is particularly useful in cases where pain and swelling radiate from the lower joints towards the higher joints.

3. Benzoic acid: This remedy is suitable for individuals with strong odor in urine or prone to kidney stones along with symptoms of gout. The joints may be swollen, stiff and extremely painful, with a feeling of dislocation.

Understanding the concept of individualized treatment:

One of the basic principles of homeopathy is individualized treatment. Rather than focusing solely on the symptoms of gout, a qualified homeopath considers a person's entire health profile. This includes not only physical symptoms but also emotional and mental aspects. By gaining a comprehensive understanding of a person's unique constitution, a homeopath can recommend remedies that address underlying imbalances and promote long-term healing.

Consultation with a qualified homeopath and tips for self-care:

While homeopathy offers a large number of potential gout remedies, it is important to consult a qualified homeopath to ensure a personalized and appropriate treatment. A homeopathic doctor will perform a thorough examination, taking into account your medical history, lifestyle factors and specific symptoms. He will then prescribe remedial measures tailored to your individual needs and monitor your progress over time.

In addition to professional guidance, there are self-care practices that can complement homeopathic gout treatment. These include adopting a gout-friendly diet, staying well hydrated, managing stress, maintaining a healthy weight, and incorporating gentle exercise into your routine. These lifestyle changes can promote the effectiveness of homeopathic remedies and contribute to overall well-being.

Conclusion:

Homeopathy offers a unique and holistic approach to managing the symptoms of gout, addressing the individual nature of the disease and tailoring medicines to each person's specific needs. By adopting the principles of "like cures like" and considering the individual's entire health profile, homeopathy aims to restore balance, relieve pain and promote overall well-being.

While homeopathic remedies can be effective in managing gout symptoms, it is important to consult a qualified homeopath for individualized advice and treatment. A professional homeopath will perform a thorough examination and prescribe medications that match your specific symptoms, triggers, and overall health.

In conjunction with homeopathic treatment, self-medication plays an important role in managing gout. Adopting a gout-friendly diet, staying well hydrated, managing stress, maintaining a healthy weight, and incorporating gentle exercise into your routine can all contribute to the effectiveness of homeopathic remedies and promote overall well-being.

It is important to remember that homeopathy, like any medical approach, requires patience and consistency. Results may vary from person to person, and it may take time to find the most appropriate drug or combination of drugs for your specific needs. Regular check-ups with your homeopath will allow adjustments to your treatment plan and provide ongoing support and guidance.

By embracing the principles of homeopathy, seeking the expertise of a qualified homeopath, and integrating self-care practices, you can be on your way to naturally managing your gout symptoms and promoting long-term health. Empower yourself with knowledge, explore the subtle healing potential of homeopathy and discover a holistic approach to finding relief from gout.

Chapter 11:

Healing Properties of Apple Cider Vinegar for Gout

In this chapter, we delve into the fascinating world of apple cider vinegar and its potential healing properties in the treatment of gout. Apple cider vinegar has long been touted for its numerous health benefits, and its role in relieving gout symptoms has received considerable attention. By understanding its potential benefits, researching its role in treating gout, and learning different ways to incorporate it into your daily routine, you can harness the power of this natural remedy to find relief. However, it is important to be aware of potential precautions and side effects to ensure safe and effective use.

An Overview of Apple Cider Vinegar and Its Potential Benefits:

Apple cider vinegar is a fermented liquid made from crushed apples. It contains acetic acid and other beneficial compounds such as vitamins, minerals and antioxidants. These ingredients contribute to its potential health benefits. When it comes to gout, apple cider vinegar is thought to help reduce inflammation, balance pH levels, and help dissolve uric acid crystals, the primary culprit behind gout attacks.

Investigating its role in treating gout symptoms:

Apple cider vinegar can potentially provide relief from gout symptoms in several ways. First, it can help alkalize the body, which can counteract the acidic conditions that contribute to gout flare-ups. By promoting a more alkaline environment, it can help reduce inflammation and prevent uric acid crystallization. Additionally, the anti-inflammatory properties of apple cider vinegar can help reduce the pain and swelling associated with gout attacks. While research is ongoing, many individuals have reported positive experiences and improvement in gout symptoms with the use of apple cider vinegar.

Different ways to incorporate apple cider vinegar into your daily routine:

There are several ways to incorporate apple cider vinegar into your daily routine to take advantage of its potential gout relief benefits. One simple method is to dilute one to two tablespoons of apple cider vinegar in a glass of warm water and consume it daily. You can also add a teaspoon or two of raw, unfiltered apple cider vinegar to herbal teas or incorporate it into homemade salad dressings or marinades for added tangy flavor. Another popular method is to make an apple cider vinegar tonic by combining it with honey and water. Experiment with different recipes and find a way that suits your taste preferences.

Precautions and potential side effects:

While apple cider vinegar may offer potential benefits for treating gout, it is essential to exercise caution and be aware of potential side effects. The acidity of apple cider vinegar can damage tooth enamel, so it is advisable to rinse your mouth with water after consuming it. In addition, excessive consumption or undiluted apple cider vinegar can lead to digestive problems or interactions with certain medications. It's important to consult with your healthcare provider before incorporating apple cider vinegar into your routine, especially if you have an underlying medical condition or are taking medication.

Conclusion:

Apple cider vinegar has gained popularity as a natural remedy for managing gout symptoms, offering potential benefits such as reducing inflammation, balancing pH levels, and helping to dissolve uric acid crystals. By incorporating apple cider vinegar into your daily routine in a safe and controlled way, you can use its potential healing properties to find relief from gout attacks. Be sure to keep precautions, potential side effects in mind, and check with your healthcare provider before making any significant changes to your gout treatment plan. With knowledge and careful use, apple cider vinegar can be a valuable tool on your journey to gout relief and better well-being.

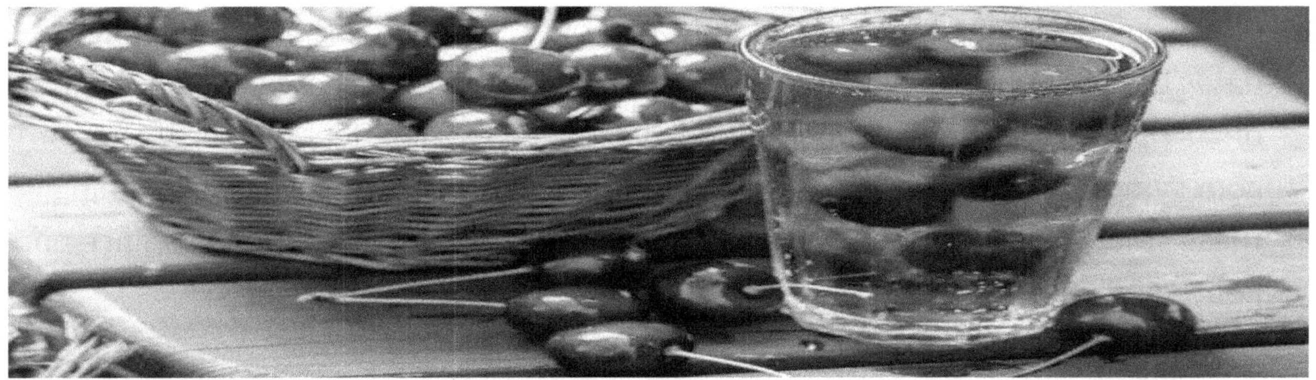

Chapter 12:

Cherry Juice and Gout: Does It Really Help?

In the realm of natural gout remedies, few have garnered as much attention as cherry juice. Many people swear by its ability to reduce the pain and inflammation associated with gout flare-ups. But does cherry juice really live up to its reputation? In this chapter, we delve into the fascinating world of cherry juice and its potential benefits in treating gout. We will explore the association between tart cherry juice and gout relief, analyze the scientific evidence supporting its effectiveness, explore potential mechanisms of its benefits, and provide recommendations for incorporating tart cherry juice into a comprehensive gout treatment plan.

Examining Connections:

Cherry juice has long been associated with gout relief, and anecdotal evidence dates back centuries. However, in recent years, scientific research has shed light on its potential effectiveness. Studies have looked at the effect of cherry juice on gout symptoms, including pain, inflammation and uric acid levels. By examining these studies, we can better understand the connection between cherry juice and gout relief.

Analysis of the scientific evidence:

Scientific research has revealed promising results regarding the potential benefits of cherry juice in the treatment of gout. Several studies have shown that consuming tart cherry juice can reduce the frequency of gout attacks and reduce the severity of symptoms. These studies used a variety of methods, including randomized controlled trials and observational studies, to assess the effect of cherry juice on gout. By analyzing the scientific evidence, we can assess the effectiveness of cherry juice as a complementary approach to the treatment of gout.

Exploring potential mechanisms:

While the exact mechanisms behind tart cherry juice's gout benefits are not yet fully understood, researchers have proposed several theories. One hypothesis suggests that tart cherry juice's anti-inflammatory properties, attributed to its high antioxidant and polyphenol content, contribute to its effectiveness in reducing gout symptoms. In addition, cherry juice may affect uric acid levels and metabolism, potentially reducing the risk of crystallization and deposition in the joints. By exploring these potential mechanisms, we can gain insight into how cherry juice exerts its beneficial effects on gout.

Recommendations for adding cherry juice:

If you're considering incorporating tart cherry juice into your gout treatment plan, there are a few factors to keep in mind. First, it is important to consult with your healthcare provider before making any significant changes to your treatment regimen. They can provide personalized advice based on your individual health profile and any potential drug interactions. Additionally, it's important to choose pure, unsweetened cherry juice to maximize its potential benefits. Consider starting with a small amount and gradually increasing your intake to gauge your body's response.

To incorporate tart cherry juice into your gout treatment plan, you can consume it as a standalone drink or incorporate it into smoothies or other recipes. It is worth noting that cherry juice should be seen as a complementary approach and not as a separate treatment. It is most effective when combined with a comprehensive gout management strategy that includes dietary changes, lifestyle modifications, and any prescribed medications.

Conclusion:

Cherry juice has emerged as a popular home remedy for gout relief, and scientific research supports its potential effectiveness. By examining the link between tart cherry juice and gout relief, analyzing the scientific evidence, exploring potential mechanisms, and providing recommendations for its inclusion, we shed light on the potential benefits of tart cherry juice in the treatment of gout. Remember that it is essential to approach cherry juice as part of a holistic approach to treating gout, in conjunction with medical advice, dietary modifications and lifestyle changes. By incorporating cherry juice into your gout treatment plan, you can potentially find relief and take the next step toward a healthier, pain-free life.

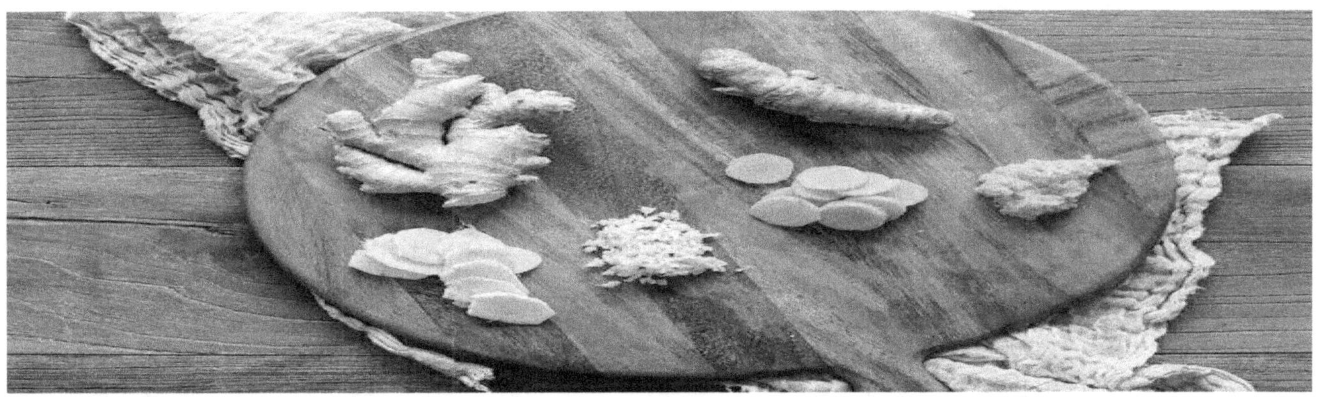

Chapter 13:

Turmeric and Ginger in Gout: Spices for Health

In this chapter, we delve into the wonderful world of turmeric and ginger, two aromatic spices known for their bright flavor and powerful medicinal properties. In addition to their culinary uses, these golden treasures have long been celebrated for their anti-inflammatory properties, making them valuable allies in the treatment of gout. Join us as we explore the many benefits of turmeric and ginger, learn how to incorporate them into our meals and drinks, and discover precautions and considerations for using this spice effectively.

Understanding Turmeric and Ginger

Turmeric, a deep yellow spice derived from the Curcuma longa plant, has been used for centuries in Ayurvedic and traditional medicine for its therapeutic properties. Curcumin, the active ingredient in turmeric, has powerful anti-inflammatory and antioxidant effects, making it a promising natural remedy for gout. Ginger, on the other hand, comes from the Zingiber officinale plant and is known for its spicy, warm flavor. Gingerol, the primary bioactive compound in ginger, has similar anti-inflammatory properties to curcumin, making it a valuable addition to our gout arsenal.

Potential benefits for the treatment of gout

Both turmeric and ginger offer a number of potential benefits when it comes to managing gout. Their anti-inflammatory properties can help reduce the swelling, redness, and pain associated with gout flare-ups. These spices can also inhibit the production of inflammatory molecules, reducing overall inflammation in the body. In addition, turmeric and ginger are thought to have antioxidant properties that can help neutralize free radicals and protect the body's cells from oxidative damage.

Methods of Incorporating Turmeric and Ginger

Incorporating turmeric and ginger into your foods and drinks is a wonderful and creative way to tap into their healing potential. Turmeric can be added to curries, stews and rice dishes, giving them a bright yellow hue and a distinct earthy flavor. Golden Milk, a traditional Ayurvedic drink made from turmeric, milk and spices, is a soothing and nourishing option for gout relief. As for ginger, it can be grated or chopped and used in stir-fries, soups and marinades to add a spicy kick. Ginger tea, made by steeping fresh ginger in hot water, offers a soothing and invigorating drink that can be enjoyed throughout the day.

Precautions and Considerations

While turmeric and ginger are generally safe to consume, there are some precautions and considerations to be aware of. If you have an underlying medical condition or are taking medication, it is recommended that you consult your healthcare provider before incorporating large amounts of these spices into your diet. Turmeric and ginger can interact with certain medications, such as blood thinners, so it is essential to seek professional advice. In addition, excessive consumption of turmeric or ginger can cause digestive problems in some individuals. Start with small amounts and gradually increase as tolerated to minimize any side effects.

Conclusion:

Turmeric and ginger are not only culinary specialties, but also powerful allies in the treatment of gout. Their anti-inflammatory properties and numerous health benefits make them valuable additions to our daily routine. By incorporating this spice into our food and drinks, we can improve the taste of our food while promoting gout relief. However, it is important to exercise caution, especially if you have specific medical conditions or are taking medication. By understanding the potential benefits and practicing moderation, you can harness the healing potential of turmeric and ginger and spice up your journey to better health.

Chapter 14:

The Magic of Epsom Salts for Gout Pain Relief

In our search for effective and natural remedies for gout pain relief, we turn our attention to a seemingly humble but remarkable mineral compound: Epsom salt. Known for its therapeutic properties, Epsom salt has been used for centuries to relieve various ailments, including gout. In this chapter, we'll delve into the role of Epsom salt in gout relief, exploring its potential benefits, various application methods, and safety considerations.

Understanding the Role of Epsom Salts in Treating Gout:

Epsom salt, scientifically known as magnesium sulfate, is a crystalline substance composed of magnesium, sulfur, and oxygen. When dissolved in water, it releases magnesium and sulfate ions that can be absorbed by the skin. Magnesium is a vital mineral that plays a key role in over 300 enzymatic reactions in the body. Sulfate, on the other hand, is known for its detoxifying properties and ability to support healthy joint function.

Exploring its potential benefits for reducing pain and inflammation:

Epsom salt is believed to offer several benefits in the treatment of gout, primarily due to its ability to reduce pain and inflammation. When used in baths or compresses, Epsom salt is thought to help draw out toxins, reduce swelling, and soothe aching joints affected by gout. The high magnesium content in Epsom salt is thought to have a muscle-relaxing effect, which can provide additional relief to gout sufferers.

Different ways to use Epsom salt baths or compresses for gout relief:

1. Epsom Salt Baths: One of the most common and enjoyable ways to use Epsom salt for gout relief is in a soothing bath. Simply fill a tub with warm water and add a cup or two of Epsom salts. Soak in the bath for 20 to 30 minutes to allow magnesium and sulfate ions to penetrate the skin and provide relief to affected joints. You can repeat this process several times a week or as needed.

2. Epsom salt compresses: For targeted relief, Epsom salt compresses can be applied directly to the affected joint. Dissolve a tablespoon of Epsom salt in a bowl of warm water. Soak a clean cloth or towel in the solution, squeeze out the excess liquid and apply to the affected area. Leave the compress on for 15 to 20 minutes to allow the minerals to absorb into the skin. Repeat as needed throughout the day.

Precautions and considerations when using Epsom salt:

While Epsom salt is generally considered safe for topical use, it is important to exercise caution and consider a few safety precautions:

1. Consult a healthcare professional: Before incorporating Epsom salt into your gout treatment plan, it is recommended to consult a healthcare professional, especially if you have any underlying medical conditions or are taking medication.

2. Allergies and skin sensitivity: Some individuals may have an allergy or skin sensitivity to Epsom salt. It is recommended to perform a patch test by applying a small amount of Epsom salt solution to a small area of skin and observing for any adverse reactions.

3. Hydration: Epsom salt baths can be relaxing and induce sweating, which can lead to dehydration. To maintain adequate hydration, it is essential to drink plenty of water before and after bathing.

4. Avoid open wounds or broken skin: Do not use Epsom salt on open wounds or broken skin as it can cause irritation or stinging sensations.

5. Use Epsom Salt Modestly: While Epsom salt baths and compresses can provide relief, it's important not to overuse them. Excessive use of Epsom salt can lead to skin dryness or potential electrolyte imbalance. It is recommended to follow recommended dosage and frequency guidelines provided by healthcare professionals or reputable sources.

6. Medical Conditions and Medications: If you have an underlying medical condition such as kidney disease or diabetes, or if you are taking medication, it is important that you consult a healthcare practitioner before using Epsom salt. They can give you personalized advice based on your specific health circumstances and help you determine if Epsom salt is right for you.

7. Pregnancy and breast-feeding: People who are pregnant or breast-feeding should exercise caution when using Epsom salt. It is recommended to consult a healthcare practitioner to assess the safety and suitability of using Epsom salt during this period.

8. Children and the Elderly: When considering the use of Epsom salt for children or the elderly, it is important to exercise caution and consult a healthcare practitioner. Dosage, frequency and application methods may need to be adjusted to ensure safety and efficacy.

Conclusion:

Epsom salt, containing magnesium and sulfate, shows promise as a natural remedy for gout pain relief. By understanding its role and potential benefits, individuals with gout can explore using Epsom salt baths or compresses as complementary approaches to their treatment plan. However, it is essential to exercise caution, follow safety precautions and consult with healthcare professionals to ensure its proper use and avoid potential complications. With the right knowledge and responsible application, Epsom salt can be a valuable tool on your journey to finding relief from gout pain and inflammation.

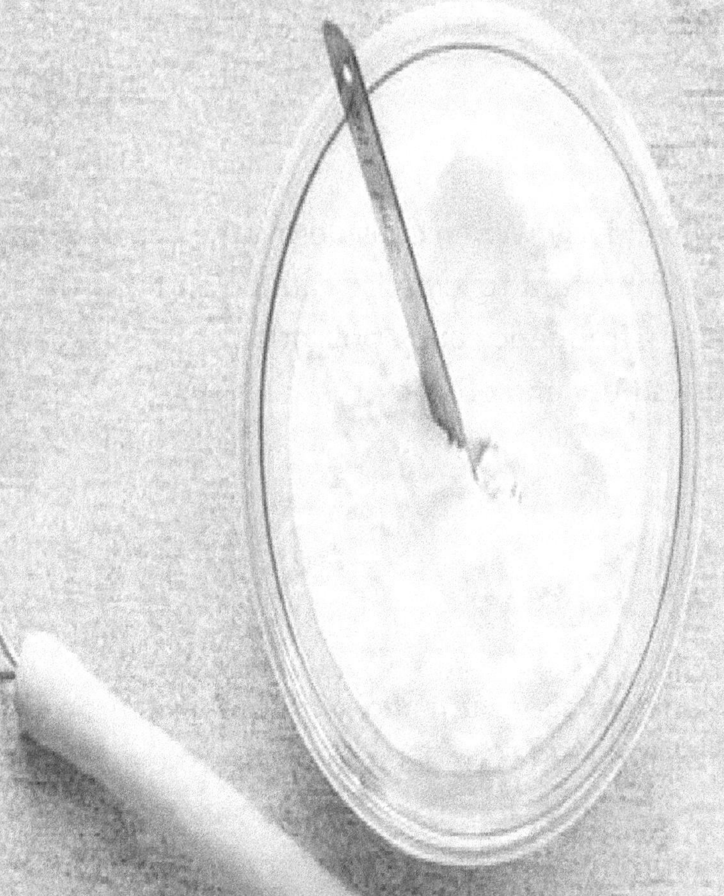

Chapter 15:

Baking Soda and Gout: Simple Kitchen Remedies for Pain

In an effort to uncover the healing potential of kitchen remedies for gout, we now turn our attention to a humble ingredient that holds remarkable promise: baking soda. Known for its versatility in cooking and cleaning, baking soda has also gained attention for its potential to provide relief from gout symptoms. In this chapter, we will delve into the fascinating world of baking soda as a home remedy for gout and explore its effectiveness, mechanisms of action, directions for use, as well as possible risks and precautions.

Understanding the use of baking soda for gout symptoms:

Baking soda, also known as sodium bicarbonate, is a white crystalline powder with alkaline properties. It has been used for centuries in a variety of applications, including as an antacid and leavening agent in baking. However, its potential benefits extend beyond the kitchen. When it comes to gout, baking soda is believed to work by changing the body's pH levels and reducing the production of uric acid.

Investigating potential mechanisms of its effectiveness:

The effectiveness of baking soda in relieving gout can be attributed to its alkalizing properties. Gout occurs when uric acid crystals build up in the joints, leading to inflammation and pain. When ingested, baking soda increases the alkalinity of the blood and urine, which can help dissolve uric acid crystals and prevent them from building up in the joints. By reducing the concentration of uric acid, baking soda aims to ease gout symptoms and provide relief.

Directions for using baking soda as a home remedy for gout:

If you're considering using baking soda as a home remedy for gout, it's important to follow some rules to ensure safety and maximize its potential benefits. Here are some recommendations to keep in mind:

1. Consult a healthcare professional: Before incorporating baking soda into your gout treatment plan, it's important to consult a healthcare professional, especially if you have an underlying medical condition or are taking medication. They can provide you with personalized advice based on your specific situation.

2. Start small: Start by taking a small amount of baking soda dissolved in water. A commonly recommended dose is half a teaspoon of baking soda mixed with a glass of water. Increase the dose gradually if necessary, but always follow the instructions of your healthcare provider.

3. Timing is key: It is generally recommended to take baking soda on an empty stomach or at least two hours after a meal. This helps avoid interference with the digestive process and allows the baking soda to have a more targeted effect.

4. Watch your body's reaction: Pay attention to how your body reacts to baking soda. While some individuals may experience relief from gout symptoms, others may not find it as effective. If you experience any adverse reactions or worsening of symptoms, discontinue use and consult your healthcare provider.

Possible risks and precautions associated with using baking soda:

While baking soda can be a useful home remedy for gout, it is important to be aware of the potential risks and take the necessary precautions. Here are some considerations to keep in mind:

1. Sodium intake: Baking soda is high in sodium, and excessive sodium intake can lead to fluid retention and high blood pressure. If you follow a low-sodium diet or have high blood pressure, it is essential to discuss the use of baking soda with your healthcare provider to ensure it is consistent with your dietary needs.

2. Drug Interactions: Baking soda can interact with certain medications such as blood pressure medications, diuretics, and others. It is important to tell your healthcare provider about all medications you are taking to avoid possible interactions. Your healthcare provider can assess the compatibility of baking soda with your current medications and adjust your treatment plan accordingly.

3. Kidney function: Baking soda can affect individuals with impaired kidney function. It is important to consult your healthcare provider if you have a history of kidney disease or if you are undergoing dialysis. They can provide instructions on how to use baking soda properly and monitor its effect on your kidney health.

4. Potential for Electrolyte Imbalance: Baking soda can alter the body's electrolyte balance, especially potassium and calcium levels. This imbalance can have consequences for individuals with certain medical conditions, such as heart disease or those taking specific medications. It is essential to discuss the use of baking soda with your healthcare provider to make sure it does not affect electrolyte levels.

5. Avoid Overconsumption: While baking soda can provide relief from gout symptoms, it is important to use it in moderation. Excessive consumption of baking soda can lead to metabolic alkalosis, a condition characterized by an imbalance of acid-base levels in the body. This can result in symptoms such as nausea, vomiting, muscle twitching and even difficulty breathing. Always follow the recommended dosage and seek medical attention in case of any side effects.

Conclusion:

Baking soda offers a simple and readily available home remedy for gout symptoms. Its alkalizing properties and potential to lower uric acid levels make it an attractive choice for those looking for natural alternatives. However, it is important to approach its use with caution, follow the instructions and consult with your healthcare professional to ensure it is appropriate for your particular circumstances.

By understanding the mechanisms of action of baking soda, following the appropriate directions for use, and being aware of potential risks and precautions, you can confidently incorporate baking soda into your gout treatment plan. Remember, the goal is to find a personalized approach that integrates both natural remedies and medical advice to effectively manage your gout symptoms and improve your overall well-being.

As with any treatment option, it's important to listen to your body, monitor your symptoms, and maintain open communication with your healthcare provider. Together, you can determine the most appropriate course of action and navigate the path to gout relief, step by step.

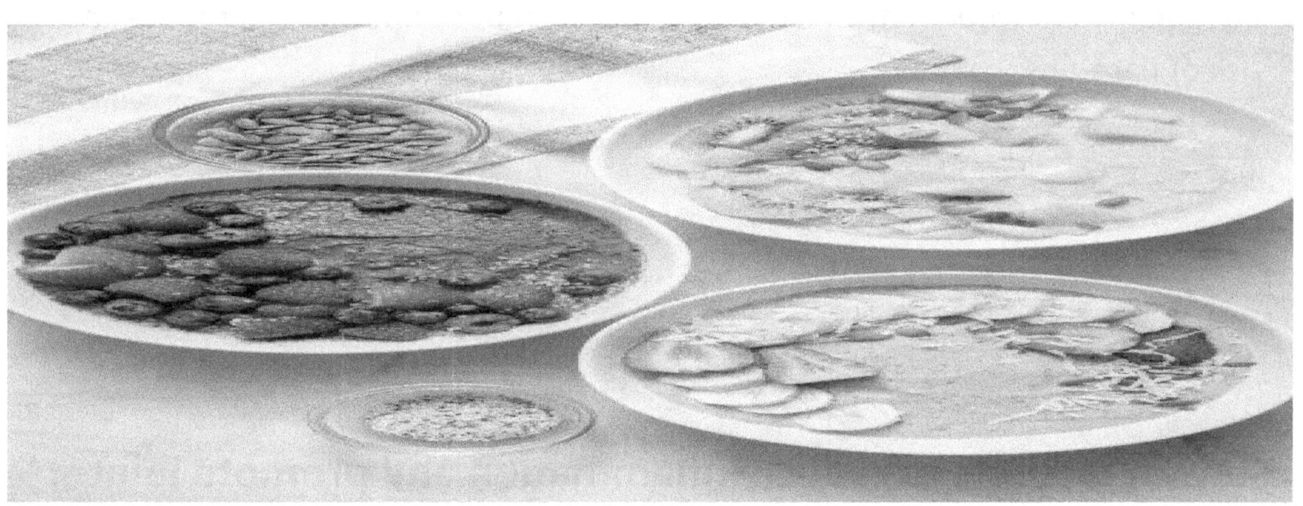

Chapter 16:

How to Make a Gout-Friendly Smoothie at Home

Smoothies are a nice and refreshing way to nourish our bodies and can also play a significant role in treating gout. In this chapter, we'll delve into the world of gout smoothies, explore their benefits, discuss key ingredients for reducing inflammation and promoting joint health, provide you with delicious recipes and variations, and offer tips for incorporating smoothies into your gout treatment plan.

A gout-friendly smoothie serves as a nutritional powerhouse that packs essential vitamins, minerals and antioxidants into a convenient and easily digestible form. They offer a practical and delicious way to incorporate anti-inflammatory ingredients into your diet, which can help ease gout symptoms and reduce the risk of flare-ups.

Key ingredients to reduce inflammation and promote joint health:

When making smoothies for gout, it's important to focus on ingredients that have anti-inflammatory properties and can support joint health. Here are some key components to consider:

1. Dark leafy greens: Spinach, kale and Swiss chard are excellent choices as they are rich in vitamins, minerals and antioxidants. They also contain high levels of chlorophyll, which can aid in detoxification.

2. Berries: Blueberries, strawberries, raspberries and cherries are full of antioxidants, especially anthocyanins, which have anti-inflammatory properties. These fruits can help neutralize free radicals and reduce inflammation in the body.

3. Pineapple: This tropical fruit contains bromelain, an enzyme known for its anti-inflammatory effects. Bromelain can help reduce the pain and swelling associated with gout.

4. Turmeric: Known for its powerful anti-inflammatory properties, turmeric contains curcumin, which has been studied for its potential to reduce inflammation and relieve gout symptoms. Including a teaspoon of turmeric in your smoothies can provide a beneficial boost.

5. Ginger: Ginger has strong anti-inflammatory and analgesic properties, making it a valuable ingredient for gout-friendly smoothies. Its unique taste will give your creations a pleasant twist.

6. Flaxseeds: Rich in omega-3 fatty acids, flaxseeds can help reduce inflammation in the body. They are also a great source of fiber, which can support healthy digestion.

Recipes and variations of smoothies for gout:

Now let's take a look at some delicious gout smoothie recipes and variations that include these key ingredients:

1. Berry Blast Smoothie:

- 1 cup spinach

- 1 cup mixed forest fruit (blueberries, strawberries, raspberries)

- 1 small banana

- 1 tablespoon of flax seeds

- 1 cup of almond milk or coconut water

2. Tropical Turmeric:

- 1 cup of cabbage

- 1 cup of pineapple chunks

- 1 small banana

- 1 teaspoon of turmeric powder

- 1 teaspoon of grated ginger

- 1 cup of coconut water

3. Green Ginger Zing:

- 1 cup Swiss chard

- 1 small cucumber

- 1 green apple

- 1 teaspoon of grated ginger

- Juice of 1 lemon

- 1 cup of filtered water

Feel free to experiment with these recipes and adjust the ingredients to suit your taste preferences. You can also add a handful of ice cubes to keep your smoothie chilled and refreshing.

Tips for incorporating smoothies into your gout treatment plan:

To get the full benefits of smoothies for gout, here are some tips to help you incorporate them into your gout treatment plan:

1. Start your day with a smoothie: Enjoying a gout-friendly smoothie in the morning can ensure a healthy and nutritious start to your day. It sets the tone for making conscious food choices and nourishing your body from the very beginning.

2. Experiment with ingredients: Don't be afraid to get creative with your smoothie recipes. Experiment with different combinations of fruits, vegetables and superfoods to find flavors you like. Variety is key to ensuring intake of a wide range of nutrients.

3. Include a source of protein: While fruits and vegetables are important ingredients in gout smoothies, it is also beneficial to include a source of protein. Adding ingredients like Greek yogurt, almond butter, or a scoop of protein powder can help stabilize your blood sugar and keep you feeling full and satisfied.

4. Watch the sugar content: Be aware of the sugar content of your smoothies, especially if you use sweet fruits. While natural sugars are generally healthier than processed sugars, it's still important to limit your intake. To balance the sweetness, consider using low-sugar fruits or incorporating vegetables such as cucumber or celery.

5. Choose homemade over store-bought: While store-bought smoothies may seem convenient, they often contain added sugars, preservatives, and artificial ingredients. Making your own smoothies at home gives you full control over the ingredients and ensures you're consuming a healthier option.

6. Pay attention to portion sizes: While smoothies can be a great way to increase your nutrient intake, it's important to consume them in moderation. A smoothie can still be high in calories, especially if you add high-calorie ingredients like nut butters or avocado. Consider using smaller portions or splitting the smoothie into two servings so you can enjoy it throughout the day.

7. Include smoothies as a snack or meal replacement: Gout smoothies can be enjoyed as a snack between meals or as a replacement for a less healthy meal. They provide a convenient and nutrient-rich alternative to processed snacks or fast food.

8. Listen to your body: Everyone's dietary needs and tolerances are unique. Pay attention to how your body reacts to the different ingredients in your smoothies. If you notice any side effects or increased gout symptoms, adjust ingredients accordingly or consult a healthcare practitioner.

Remember, gout-friendly smoothies are only one piece of the gout treatment puzzle. They should be part of a comprehensive approach that includes a balanced diet, regular exercise, hydration, and appropriate medications if prescribed by your healthcare provider.

By incorporating these tips and embracing the power of gout smoothies, you can nourish your body, reduce inflammation, and support your overall gout treatment plan. Hooray for a tasty and healthy journey!

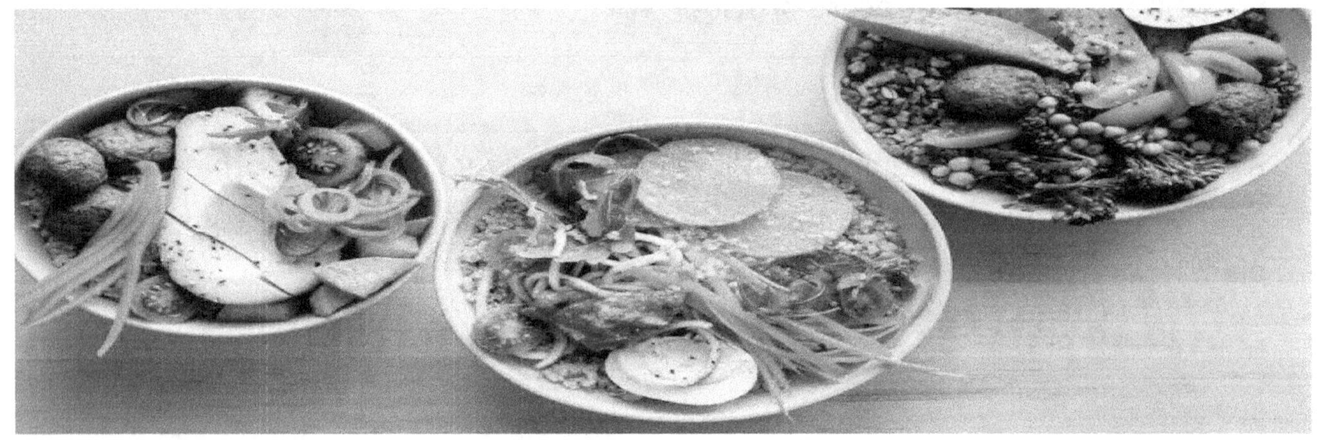

Chapter 17:

Gout Meal Planning: Recipes and Ideas for Healthy Eating

In this chapter, we delve into the world of gout meal planning, exploring strategies, recipes, and nutritional considerations that support effective gout management. By carefully choosing daily meals, we can significantly reduce the frequency and intensity of gout attacks, thereby supporting overall joint health and well-being. With a focus on taste, variety and nutritional balance, we want to help you create a sustainable and enjoyable gout-friendly diet.

Strategies for meal planning for gout:

Effective meal planning is essential when it comes to managing your day. By strategically choosing ingredients and structuring meals, we can optimize our nutritional intake while minimizing the risk of triggering gout attacks. Here are some key strategies to keep in mind:

1. Include low-purine foods: Purines contribute to the production of uric acid, so it is essential to include low-purine foods in your diet. Choose lean proteins like chicken, turkey, and fish, and favor plant-based protein sources like beans, lentils, and tofu.

2. Eat fruits and vegetables: Fruits and vegetables are rich in essential vitamins, minerals and antioxidants, while also being low in purines. They should form the basis of your gout-friendly meals. Aim for a brightly colored variety to maximize the range of nutrients.

3. Choose whole grains: Whole grains like brown rice, quinoa, and whole grain bread are excellent choices for treating gout. They provide fiber and essential nutrients while minimizing the risk of blood sugar spikes.

4. Limit high-purine foods: While it's important to focus on low-purine options, it's also important to limit high-purine foods, such as organ meats, shellfish, and certain types of fish (eg, anchovies, sardines). . Eating these foods in moderation can help reduce the risk of gout flare-ups.

Recipe ideas below:

Now let's look at some gout-friendly recipes that you can incorporate into your diet. From satisfying breakfast options to delicious lunch and dinner ideas, these recipes are designed to delight your taste buds while supporting your gout goals.

1. Breakfast:

   - Vegetable omelette with spinach, peppers and mushrooms

   - One-day oats with mixed fruit and a sprinkling of chopped walnuts

   - Avocado toast on whole wheat bread topped with cherry tomatoes and a drizzle of olive oil

2. Lunch:

   - Quinoa salad with grilled chicken, cucumbers, cherry tomatoes and lemon vinaigrette

   - Lentil soup with a side of mixed green salad and lemon-tahini dressing

   - Grilled salmon with steamed asparagus and quinoa pilaf

3. Dinner:

   - Roasted chicken breast with roasted Brussels sprouts and sweet potatoes

   - Prawns stir-fried with a colorful mixture of peppers, chips and broccoli served with brown rice

   - Zucchini noodles (zoodles) with turkey meatballs and homemade marinara sauce

4. Snacks:

   - Greek yogurt with a handful of mixed berries and a sprinkling of chia seeds

   - Celery sticks with almond butter and raisins

   - Roasted chickpeas flavored with paprika and cumin

Nutritional considerations and recommendations:

When planning meals for gout, it is important to pay attention to certain nutritional factors:

1. Hydration: Stay adequately hydrated by drinking water throughout the day. Proper hydration helps flush out uric acid and supports kidney function.

2. Fiber: Include foods high in fiber, such as fruits, vegetables, whole grains, and legumes, to promote healthy digestion and maintain an optimal weight. Fiber also helps regulate blood sugar levels and can contribute to a feeling of fullness, preventing overeating.

3. Omega-3 fatty acids: Include foods rich in omega-3 fatty acids, such as fatty fish (salmon, mackerel, sardines), flax seeds and chia seeds. These healthy fats have anti-inflammatory properties and can help reduce the inflammation associated with gout.

4. Limit saturated and trans fats: Avoid or minimize consumption of foods high in saturated and trans fats, such as fatty meats, fried foods, processed snacks, and commercially available baked goods. These fats can increase inflammation and worsen gout symptoms.

5. Moderate alcohol intake: Excessive alcohol consumption can increase the risk of gout flare-ups. If you choose to drink, do so in moderation and choose lower purine options such as light beer or moderate amounts of wine.

Creating a sustainable and enjoyable gout diet:

Adopting a gout-friendly diet shouldn't be seen as restrictive or boring. Instead, it's an opportunity to explore new flavors, experiment with nutritious ingredients, and discover the joy of nourishing your body. Here are some tips to help you create a sustainable and enjoyable gout-friendly diet:

1. Experiment with herbs and spices: Use herbs and spices liberally in your cooking to add flavor and depth to your dishes. Turmeric, ginger, basil, oregano, and cinnamon are just a few examples of tasty options that also offer potential anti-inflammatory benefits.

2. Embrace Meal Prep: Set aside time each week to plan and prepare meals in advance. This can help you make healthier choices and avoid using convenience foods, which can be high in purines and unhealthy fats.

3. Get creative with substitutions: Look for creative ways to swap out high-purine ingredients in your favorite recipes. Instead of regular rice, use cauliflower rice, for example, or choose zucchini noodles instead of pasta.

4. Enjoy different cuisines: Explore different cuisines that naturally contain gout-friendly ingredients. Mediterranean, Japanese, and vegetarian/vegan diets often contain large amounts of fruits, vegetables, whole grains, and legumes.

5. Find support: Connect with others who are also managing gout or looking for gout-friendly meal ideas. Online forums, support groups, or even cooking classes can provide a sense of community and inspiration on your journey.

Remember, gout meal planning is not about deprivation or strict rules. It's about making informed choices, fueling your body with healthy ingredients and finding a balance that works for you. By adopting a gout-friendly diet, you can experience relief from gout symptoms while enjoying delicious, satisfying foods that support your overall health and well-being.

So let's embark on this culinary adventure as we explore the delicious world of gout-friendly recipes and meal ideas. Get ready to tantalize your taste buds, nourish your body and take control of your gout treatment with delicious and nutritious meals.

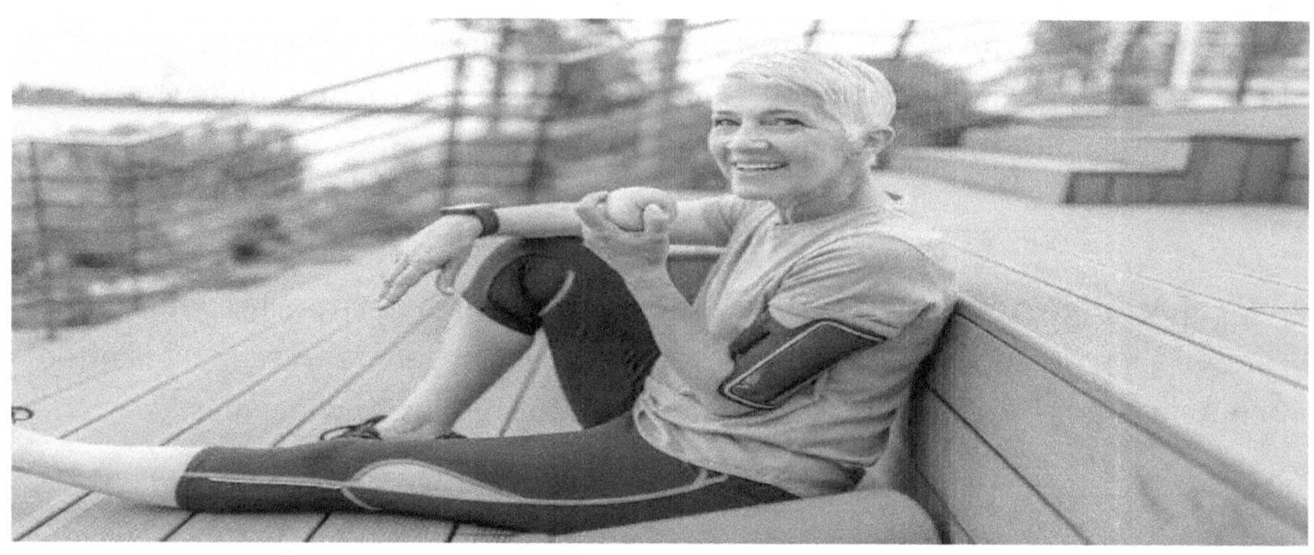

Chapter 18:

Lifestyle Changes for Long-Term Gout Management

In this final chapter of "The Complete Guide to Home Remedies for Gout: From Kitchen to Cure," we delve into the critical role of long-term lifestyle changes in effectively managing gout. While home remedies and natural treatments are invaluable tools, it is a consistent commitment to healthier choices that ultimately leads to lasting relief and improved quality of life. This chapter highlights the importance of adopting and maintaining these lifestyle changes, providing strategies, tips and resources to support your journey to long-term gout management.

Emphasizing the importance of long-term lifestyle changes:

Gout is a chronic condition and managing its symptoms requires a holistic approach that goes beyond quick fixes. By making long-term lifestyle changes, you can address the underlying factors contributing to gout flare-ups, minimize their occurrence, and promote overall health and well-being.

Strategies for managing stress and improving sleep quality:

Stress and lack of sleep are associated with an increased incidence of gout. In this section, we'll explore effective strategies for managing stress and improving sleep quality. From mindfulness techniques and relaxation exercises to creating healthy sleep habits, you'll discover practical approaches to reducing stress levels and promoting restorative sleep. By incorporating stress management and prioritizing sleep, you'll create a solid foundation for managing your day.

Tips for maintaining a healthy weight and managing comorbidities:

Maintaining a healthy weight is essential for treating gout, as excess weight can contribute to higher uric acid levels. In this section, we provide practical tips on how to achieve and maintain a healthy weight through a balanced diet and regular physical activity. You'll gain insight into portion control, careful eating practices, and the importance of incorporating low-impact exercise suitable for individuals with gout. We also discuss the importance of managing comorbidities such as high blood pressure and diabetes, as they can worsen gout symptoms. By effectively managing these conditions, you can improve your overall health and reduce the likelihood of gout flare-ups.

Resources for ongoing support and self-care for gout management:

Treating gout is a journey that requires ongoing support and self-care. This section highlights valuable resources that can help you in your long-term gout management efforts. From support groups and online communities to educational websites and trusted sources of information, you'll find a wealth of resources to help you stay informed, connected, and motivated. We also emphasize the importance of self-care practices tailored to your specific needs, including relaxation techniques, hobbies and activities that promote physical and emotional well-being.

By making long-term lifestyle changes, managing stress effectively, prioritizing sleep, maintaining a healthy weight, managing comorbidities, and utilizing available resources, you will create a comprehensive gout treatment plan. This chapter empowers you to take control of your health and take a proactive approach to treating gout. Remember that while gout may be a chronic condition, it does not define you. With commitment, persistence, and the support of a comprehensive lifestyle plan, you can experience long-term relief, improved quality of life, and a future filled with vitality.

Congratulations on completing "The Complete Guide to Home Remedies for Gout: From Kitchen to Cure". Armed with the knowledge and tools presented in this book, you are now equipped to make informed decisions and adopt a holistic approach to treating gout. With a combination of natural remedies, dietary changes, lifestyle modifications, and ongoing support, you have the power to take control of your gout and live life to the fullest. May your journey to gout relief be filled with success, empowerment and renewed vitality.

Conclusion: Getting relief from gout with home remedies

In The Complete Guide to Gout Home Remedies: From Kitchen to Cure, we've embarked on a transformative journey, exploring the realm of natural remedies and empowering you to take control of your gout treatment. Now that we're coming to the end of this comprehensive guide, let us recap the key takeaways and give you the encouragement and tools you need to incorporate home remedies into a comprehensive gout treatment plan.

Throughout this book, we shed light on the intricacies of gout, from understanding its causes and triggers to exploring the wide range of natural remedies available to you. We delved into the importance of lifestyle changes, highlighting the link between diet, exercise, hydration and gout flare-ups. By adopting a gout-friendly diet, incorporating anti-inflammatory foods, and staying adequately hydrated, you can significantly reduce the frequency and intensity of gout attacks.

We also explored the power of herbal remedies, essential oils and homeopathy, recognizing the potential of nature's healing properties to provide relief. From apple cider vinegar and cherry juice to turmeric, ginger, Epsom salt and baking soda, we've uncovered the huge potential of these common kitchen ingredients. By incorporating them into your daily routine, you can take advantage of their anti-inflammatory and pain-relieving properties to find comfort and relief from gout symptoms.

At the end of this journey, we want to encourage you to take what you've learned and apply it to your life. Treating gout is a complex and ongoing process, and incorporating home remedies into your daily routine can greatly improve your quality of life. By taking a proactive approach and making long-term lifestyle changes, you can effectively manage gout and reduce its impact on your well-being.

We want to give you the opportunity to become the driver of your own journey to health. Consult with your healthcare professionals, adapt the recommendations in this book to meet your specific needs, and make informed decisions about your gout treatment plan. By understanding the principles of each home remedy, considering potential drug interactions, and seeking guidance when needed, you can safely and confidently incorporate these natural remedies into your routine.

Remember that the road to gout relief may require patience and persistence. Each individual's experience with gout is unique, and it may take time to find the medication combination that works best for you. Be open to experimentation, monitor your symptoms and reactions, and make adjustments. If you stay committed to your health and wellness, you may find the relief you seek.

In closing, we would like to express our gratitude for joining us on this journey. We hope that "The Complete Guide to Gout Home Remedies: From Kitchen to Cure" has provided you with valuable insights, practical tips and inspiration to take control of your gout and improve your quality of life. Armed with knowledge and armed with natural remedies, you have the tools to help you navigate the complexities of the day and pave the way for a healthier, pain-free future.

Remember that you are not alone in this journey. Reach out to support networks, share your experiences, and draw strength from those who understand the challenges you face. By taking a holistic approach to treating gout, including home remedies, you can find relief, regain your vitality, and embark on a journey of greater well-being.

Now, armed with the knowledge and empowerment gained from this guide, it's time to take the first step toward living with reduced gout symptoms. Harness the power of home remedies, make informed decisions, and let this guide be your trusted companion on your journey to relief from gout. Your journey begins now.